TEACHING AUTISTIC CHILDREN TO COMMUNICATE

Paige Shaughnessy Hinerman

University of Utah
Salt Lake City

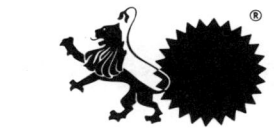

AN ASPEN PUBLICATION®
Aspen Systems Corporation
Rockville, Maryland
London
1983

Library of Congress Cataloging in Publication Data

Hinerman, Paige Shaughnessy.
Teaching autistic children to communicate.

Bibliography: p. 171. Includes index.
1. Autistic children—Treatment.
2. Communicative disorders in children.
I. Title. [DNLM: 1. Autism, Infantile—Therapy.
2. Communication. WM 203.5 H662t]
RJ506.A9H55   1983   618.92'898206   83-10016
ISBN: 0-89443-884-0

Publisher: John Marozsan
Editorial Director: R. Curtis Whitesel
Executive Managing Editor: Margot Raphael
Editorial Services: Scott Ballotin
Printing and Manufacturing: Debbie Collins

Library of Congress Catalog Card Number: 83-10016
ISBN: 0-89443-884-0

Printed in the United States of America

1   2   3   4   5

To the many autistic children
who have touched my heart
and to their parents
who trusted me and taught me compassion

Like a bungling crusader
I came screaming,
tearing at the shadows
of your universe.
From distant corners,
alien worlds,
I came poking at the secrets
of your endless motion.
Probing the echoes
of your private insulation,
I ached to break the bonds
that kept you from us.

Hope tempered with caution,
riddles solved with puzzles,
I groped for ways to set you free—
and, I nearly missed the moment
of your transformation.

When did you cease your aimless circling?
When did your course proclaim such purpose?
And, when did you retrieve the sunlight
from the shadows?
Free, now, to learn, discover, explore,
You'll struggle more than ever,
while I, oh! I will learn to wait.

Table of Contents

Preface

This manual is for people who work with autistic children. The material was developed to be used by speech clinicians, special education teachers, and therapists who are faced with the task of educating the severely autistic, noncommunicating child. The procedures are designed to give the professional a step-by-step process for teaching the uncommunicative child to communicate. The behavior management techniques are included as a necessary prerequisite for training in communication. I have attempted to present a workable synthesis of behavior therapy, communication training, and the use of manual communication. These procedures were developed and have evolved over the years; they represent the best of my experience in working with the most difficult of autistic children.

The written programs and procedures are purposely detailed, a characteristic that some may find laborious. However, I have often been disappointed by texts that fall short of their claims to present the "how to's" of teaching a skill. The detailed information and examples in this manual will, I hope, ensure against such disappointment. (The names of the children in the examples are, however, entirely fictitious; any similarity or likeness to actual individuals is unintended and coincidental.)

The emphasis of the manual is on practical experience rather than on theoretical explanations. However, it may help some readers to know the theoretical assumptions underlying the information presented. These basic assumptions may be summarized as follows:

- Behaviorism must be tempered with humanism. Behaviorism fosters the growth of the human potential. Without behaviorism, we would lose sight of the goals; without humanism, we would forget the individual worth of each handicapped child.
- Autism can be considered a psychological or an emotional disorder only in the sense that the neurological structures or processes respon-

sible for emotional and social development are nonfunctional. Autism is not the result of pathological parental attitudes.

- Until science provides us with a medical or physiological remedy, the best we can do is practice our "art" in the most scientific manner possible.
- Communication is one aspect of an intricate system of behavior that constitutes the human organism. Viewed as such, communication cannot be treated independently of other behaviors; it must be treated as a part of the dynamic interaction between organism and environment.

If anything is accomplished through this work, I hope it will be that the job of the professional is made a little more enlightened. Autism is still in its infancy as far as research and technology are concerned. I hope, however, that we will live to see the day when educational remediation is made obsolete by advances in prevention and cure. Until that day, we must be held accountable for providing educational and therapeutic programs based on sound principles and good sense. If this manual has contributed to that sense of accountability, it has achieved its purpose.

Paige S. Hinerman
September 1983

Acknowledgments

I would like to thank the friends and loved ones who cared enough to support my efforts to complete this work. I would especially like to thank my husband, who saved me the trouble of getting ulcers by doing all the worrying himself.

Chapter 1

The Nature of Autism: An Introduction

WHAT IS AUTISM?

The following four cases illustrate the characteristics of autism:

Tom

Tom's parents report that as an infant he seemed to be progressing normally until he was about 2½ years old. Though he possessed no single quality that made him stand out intellectually, he could say a few words, had passed all the developmental motor milestones that otherwise would have indicated mental retardation, and, to all those around him, he appeared to be quite normal. Suddenly, he lost all forms of communication, became unexplainably "moody" and fussy, and withdrew from social interaction of any kind.

Confused and distraught, Tom's parents sought medical help, but found no explanation for Tom's peculiar behavior. A series of psychological and educational examinations eventually led to the diagnosis of autism; and, subsequently, Tom was placed in a treatment program for behaviorally disturbed children. Prior to his educational placement, however, Tom developed several unusual behaviors, including resistance to toilet training, obsessive preoccupation with drinking straws, continual flicking of objects (usually straws) between his fingers, and (apparently) unprovoked "spells" of giggling, alternating with "spells" of whining and agitation.

Ronnie

Ronnie's mother knew that something was wrong from the moment she brought her newborn son home from the hospital. Complications at the time of birth nearly caused the death of both mother and son. Though

Ronnie did not appear to be mentally retarded or physically frail (he sat up, crawled, walked, and did other things at the normal stages, and was husky for his age), he did not use any verbal speech until he was four years old. Even when speech emerged, it was unusual in the sense that he used only a few words, used them very rarely, and used them only when he wanted something very badly. Ronnie seemed to have little interest in family members, showed little affection for anyone, avoided looking at people, did not smile, and did not play with other children. His sole interest, at various times in his first few years, was in spinning the wheels of toy trucks, watching automobile windshield wipers move back and forth, and agilely using a screwdriver to dismantle washing machines, Xerox machines and electric wall-outlet coverings. In fact, Ronnie was oblivious to dangers of any kind, which led him to climb casually onto rooftops, wander into busy streets, and play with electrical equipment.

Sherrie

Sherrie was, by all accounts, normal (though somewhat active) until about age two. At that time, she became extremely active and aggressive. She would run about the house, tipping over flower pots and breaking furniture. She rocked herself for hours at a time, refusing to come out of her little corner even for food. She was impossible to take shopping or to restaurants because she always caused a scene by screaming, destroying property, or running away. By age four, Sherrie could say a few words, but never used speech to communicate with others. Instead, she echoed the last words of what others said. When pressed to imitate, however, she would become angry and strike out at the nearest adult. Loud noises— such as clapping, noisy crowds (as in school lunchrooms), and even some kinds of music—seemed to make Sherrie fidgety.

Robert

Robert was the result of a pregnancy complicated by maternal diabetes and a difficult delivery. In the first few months of life, Robert showed signs of difficulty in feeding and sleeping. He refused to be cuddled and rejected his mother's attempts to comfort him when he cried. At about one year of age, Robert's mother became concerned about his frequent colds and ear infections. A medical examination revealed severe middle ear infection, but failed to show any hearing loss. The ear infections were corrected, but Robert continued to be "withdrawn;" he did not babble or begin to use the vocal intonation patterns that precede words, as other children do.

Robert was obsessed with the Yellow Pages of the telephone book and with the TV Guide. His mother reports that, by the time he was two years old, Robert would sit crosslegged on the floor, Yellow Pages in his lap, staring incessantly at the words on the page while flicking his fingers wildly in the air. When Robert was three years old, his mother took him to a psychiatrist, and he was subsequently enrolled in a school for disturbed children. Professionals there refused to believe the reports that Robert could "read." He was "treated" for a psychological problem—and so was his mother.

A year later, Robert's mother enrolled him in another children's program at a center for behaviorally disturbed and autistic children. Here, professionals decided to test the accuracy of the mother's accounts of Robert's reading ability. They discovered that, when asked to point to *any* word on a page or to find *any* word in the Yellow Pages, Robert could do it without hesitation. The conclusion was that, although Robert may not have fully understood the meaning of these words, he had, somehow, deciphered the phonetic code. Eventually, this unusual ability was used to bridge the communication gap. Robert was taught to point to words, then to use Scrabble letters to spell what he wanted. Robert eventually learned to use sign language and some rudimentary forms of verbal language to express his needs and wants, but he never really learned to communicate in a spontaneous or social way.

BACKGROUND

The children described above are all autistic. They are different from each other in many respects, but they all have certain characteristics in common. Most notably, these characteristics include lack of language or unusual language development and social behavior that is peculiar. For decades, educators and other professionals have argued over the exact nature of autism. They have tried to define the characteristics found in all autistic children and to isolate those that are found *only* in autism. Investigators disagree on the relevant criteria, but they all agree that the syndrome is a seriously incapacitating disorder that encompasses behaviors that set autism apart from all other disorders.

The earliest accounts of the autistic syndrome were presented by Kanner (1943), who described a group of 11 children who displayed unusual behaviors that were present from infancy and seemed to cluster in socially related or language-related peculiarities. Though earlier descriptions of children displaying autistic behaviors existed (Ritvo, 1976; Webster, 1980b; J.K. Wing, 1976), Kanner was the first person to describe the cluster of unusual behaviors that seemed to be peculiar to this group of children and to give a name to the pattern of behaviors he observed.

Prior to Kanner, the term *autism* had been used to describe a symptom of certain types of mental disorders, but it had not been applied to describe a syndrome. The term was first used by Bleuler (1913) to describe a symptom of a psychiatric disorder in connection with schizophrenia in adults. In this disorder, the patients seemed unable to relate to others, though they had, at one time or another in their lives, related normally as members of the social community. With the onset of the disorder, they withdrew or removed themselves from relationships. The failure to communicate was a manifestation of their extreme absorption in themselves.

Kanner noted that this withdrawal did not precisely fit the 11 young children he had observed, but the aloneness he observed in these children was similar to that of the patients described by Bleuler. He was convinced that, rather than choosing to withdraw from the world, these children were innately incapable of creating or responding to social relationships (Kanner, 1973). Because the affective characteristics of these children resembled those of Bleuler's patients, and because Kanner was unable to find a more suitable word to describe the illness with which these children were afflicted, he applied the term *autism* to the disorder. In an effort to accentuate the early onset of the disorder, Kanner called the syndrome *early infantile autism*.

Despite the precautions taken by Kanner in describing the syndrome, early infantile autism has been variously regarded as childhood schizophrenia (Bender, 1947), symbiotic psychosis (Mahler, 1952), atypical ego development (Rank, 1949), and childhood psychosis and emotional disturbance (Hassibi & Breuer, 1980). The choice of the term *autism* has in fact led to some confusion over the nature of the disorder. In the four decades since Kanner first described the syndrome, autistic children, and their parents, have been psychoanalyzed, psychotherapized, institutionalized, drugged, deprived of sensory stimulation, overstimulated, treated with electroshock therapy, treated with operant conditioning, put on special diets, and put on megavitamins. Somehow, the condition survives.

Disturbances of affect preoccupied the literature on autism for many years (Despert, 1968; Eisenberg, 1956; Kanner, 1943). It was not until recently that interest in language, perception, cognition, and the neurological bases of the disorder came into focus as genuine symptoms of the disorder. Kanner's description of early infantile autism involved children who were unable to develop relationships with people, who had a delay in the acquisition of speech, who failed to use speech for communicative purposes after it had developed, whose peculiarities of speech included delayed echolalia and pronoun reversal, who indulged in repetitive and stereotypic play activities, who were obsessive in their insistence on sameness, and who lacked imagination but had a good rote memory and normal physical appearance (Kanner, 1943).

Although Kanner saw the autistic child as one possessing normal or a high degree of intelligence and displaying no signs of physical handicap (Kanner, 1946), it has now come to be recognized that the disorder has many degrees of severity and as many variations of the same syndrome. Most professionals now believe that, though the term *autism* may have been an unfortunate choice for the disorder, it now serves merely as a label (Rutter, 1978a). There is nothing to be gained by trying to analyze the term. It should be recognized that the word was intended to describe the social dysfunction, one behavior in a set of several behaviors, that *describes,* rather than *defines,* the children. In recognizing this set of behaviors as a syndrome, no causal factors are implied; rather, behaviors that are universal (all autistic children have them) and specific (they are not usually found in other disorders) are described.

BEHAVIORAL CHARACTERISTICS

Many professionals, in their attempts to define autism, have emphasized one or more of the many symptoms that they believe to be the core of the disorder (Kanner, 1946; Ritvo, 1976; Rutter, 1978a; L. Wing, 1972). This indicates that, until we have a diagnostic tool that can measure autism on the basis of etiology or on the basis of some medical scale, we are dealing only with a group of behaviors; and, as long as we are dealing with a group of behaviors, there will be disagreement over the limits and boundaries of those identifying behaviors.

The behaviors that are always seen in autism are, according to Rutter (1978a), a pervasive failure to develop social relationships; language retardation, consisting of impaired comprehension, echolalia, and pronoun reversal; and ritualistic or stereotyped compulsive behavior. The National Society for Children and Adults with Autism (1980) presents a broader range of behaviors to be included in the description of autism. These behaviors include:

- slow development or lack of physical, social, and learning skills
- immature rhythms of speech, limited understanding of ideas, and use of words without the usual meaning to them
- abnormal responses to sensations (sight, hearing, touch, pain, balance, smell, taste—any one or a combination of these responses may be affected)
- abnormal ways of relating to people, objects, and events

Though these behaviors cover a variety of dysfunctions, the emphasis is on disturbances of development, language, sensory modalities, and social competence. While the list of symptoms describes which areas may be malfunctioning in the autistic child, it does not define to what extent there is a disruption of the behavior; nor does it describe the specific behaviors that indicate these areas are dysfunctional. For example, what behavior would indicate an abnormal response to sound?

The American Psychiatric Association (1980) describes autism as a pervasive developmental disorder. It lists the following categories representing abnormalities in the autistic child:

- failure to develop interpersonal relationships
- gross impairment in communicative ability
- bizarre responses to various aspects of the environment
- onset before the age of 30 months
- hallucinations, delusions, loosening of associations, and incoherence, as in schizophrenia

Though individual autistic children will display different behavioral manifestations in each of these categories, they will have abnormalities in all of them.

According to Ornitz and Ritvo (1976), autism has the following behavioral characteristics:

- perceptual disturbances
- disturbances of developmental rate
- disturbances of relating
- disturbances of speech and language
- disturbances of motility

At present, categorization of the child who may or may not be autistic is a difficult task. While some professionals adhere strictly to the criteria laid down by Kanner, others insist that the categories be extended to include new information about autism, such as organic pathology, discovered since the time of Kanner (Rutter, 1978a; Walter, Aldridge, Cooper, O'Gorman, McCallum, & Winter, 1971). Ultimately, the use of the label is important only to the researcher. There will always be children who do not fit the pattern exactly; there will always be an overlap of disorders. The label is not important in this sense: naming the disorder will not provide a cure. However, to the extent that the diagnostic label provides us with information about how certain behaviors can best be treated, and to the extent that having a diagnosis leads to the procurement of that treatment, then the label serves.

Until medical treatments are found for autism, professionals must be concerned with ensuring the most appropriate and most effective education for autistic children as early in life as possible (Fish, 1976b). While theorists speculate about the nature of autism and researchers try to decide which behaviors really constitute autism, therapists and educators are more concerned with finding ways of working with a host of behaviors that may or may not be a part of the syndrome. Different theorists have different ideas about autism. While classification remains a problem, concentration on behavioral characteristics that can be modified for the improvement of autistic children's lives is up to the therapist and the educator.

Language Impairment

The communication impairments of autistic children are discussed in detail in later chapters. However, since language impairment is one of the primary descriptors of autism, some mention of it should be made here.

Impairment of communication in autistic children consists of immature grammatical structure, delayed or immediate echolalia, pronominal reversal, nominal aphasia (inability to name objects), inability to use abstract terms, metaphorical language (utterances whose usage is idiosyncratic and whose meaning is not clear), abnormal speech melody, and, often, lack of nonverbal communication, such as socially appropriate facial expressions and gestures (Schuler & Baldwin, 1981). Autistic children have impaired prelanguage skills (Rutter, 1978b). They do not show social imitation (such as learning to wave "bye-bye"). They have difficulty understanding gestures (L. Wing, 1972), and they fail to follow instructions if cues for social context are absent (Rutter, 1972), which is indicative of poor receptive language. Unusual patterns of babbling (lacking the rich variety of normal two-year-olds) extends to unusual speech patterns, such as monotone pitch and inappropriately modulated intonation patterns. Echolalia is common among autistic children who do develop speech; however, mutism, or a kind of language that does not seem intended for the purpose of interpersonal communication, is equally common (L. Wing, 1976). In many cases, the delayed and deviant language development of autistic children is out of keeping with their intellectual level (Wetherby & Gaines, 1982). Often, autistic children fail to develop any functional communication, either verbal or nonverbal; 50 percent never gain useful speech (Rutter, 1978b).

Impaired Social Relationships

It is difficult to separate social relatedness from language development, particularly since many of the skills for both are acquired very early in life and are dependent upon each other (Webster, 1980a). Kanner noted that autistic children have a disturbance of affect (Kanner, 1943), and for many years it was assumed that the social abnormalities were responsible for the peculiar language development or for the lack of language (mutism). In discussing the irregularities of development and the disturbances of the modulation of sensory input, relatedness, and language, Ornitz and Ritvo (1976) offer the following observation:

> The notion that autistics have a primary affective deficiency which interferes with expression of their assumed normal or superior intellectual and cognitive potentials has given way to the recognition that their intellectual deficiencies are every bit as real as in patients with 'primary retardation.' (p. 16)

It is now recognized that a dysfunction of the central nervous system causes the deviant development of social relatedness (Howlin, 1978; Ritvo, 1976), including the emotional disturbances mentioned by earlier authors. Although the term *social withdrawal* may be applied to some children who seem to be progressing normally until about the second or third year, it is probably more appropriate to think of the social abnormalities of autistic children as an inability to relate to others (for whatever reasons—cognitive, linguistic, or broadly neurological). This inability to relate to others manifests itself in several ways, including avoidance of eye-to-eye gaze, inability to use the eyes or facial expressions to indicate emotion, inability to play imitative games, lack of cooperative play skills, and so on. Autistic children typically do not follow their parents about the house, imitating household chores (M.K. DeMyer, Alpern, Barton, W.E. DeMyer, Churchill, Hingtgen, Bryson, Pontius, & Kimberlin, 1972; Menolascino & Eyde, 1979); nor do they develop (or there is delayed development of) meaningful use of objects and toys, such as miniature tea sets, miniature houses, farm animals, and so on. In addition, they lack imaginative or make-believe play (Rutter, 1978a). Often, as infants, autistic babies resist being held and are not cuddly. Others may be cuddly at first, then begin to stiffen later in infancy (Everard, 1980). While many autistic children seem to be hyperactive, many are also abnormally lethargic (M.K. DeMyer, 1979).

Impaired social relationships, often viewed as the primary characteristic in early infantile autism, may show up in behavioral characteristics such as lack of responsiveness to people, lack of interest in people, failure to develop attachment to the mother (as infants), lack of eye contact and facial responsiveness, and indifference or aversion to affection and physical contact (American Psychiatric Association, 1980). Autistic children fail to develop cooperative play skills and friendships in the early years, though some may later develop attachments to certain individuals (DesLauries, 1978).

Other Abnormalities

In addition to abnormal language and social development, autistic children display unusual responses to their environment; that is, they may resist minor changes, such as the rearrangement of furniture, or they may have tantrums for hours when a favorite object is placed on the wrong shelf. They may have an obsessive attachment to certain objects, which they will insist on having with them at all times. Unlike the normal child, who may enjoy having a favorite doll or blanket to carry around, the autistic child may insist on having a piece of string, a spoon, or a drinking straw. Many autistic children have an aversion to clothing; this can have adverse effects when these children decide to "strip" in public.

Ritualistic behavior is common among autistic children. Often referred to as self-stimulatory behavior, or self-stimulation, the continuous motor movements usually involve rocking the body back and forth, or performing any number of elaborate and finely coordinated limb movements, such as arm waving, finger-flicking or tapping, spinning or twirling objects, and hand gazing. Stereotyped play patterns—such as lining things up (over and over again), spinning the wheels on toy trucks or cars, or becoming involved in other ritualistic behaviors to the exclusion of all other activities—are other examples of autistic children's unusual responses to their environment (Rutter, 1978a).

Autistic children have severe disturbances in the development of perception (Ornitz, Guthrie, & Farley, 1977; Prior, 1979). These difficulties are usually evident within the first two years of life (Rimland, 1964), and some are noticed from birth. Mothers of autistic children report that their children screamed incessantly and could be comforted only by motion (L. Wing, 1972); others report that their children were unusually flaccid, never cried, did not reach out to be picked up, or drew back from physical touch (Fish, 1978a; L. Wing, 1972). Some autistic children are excessively fearful, while others show an amazing lack of fear. Some seem not to feel pain. Some autistic children appear to be deaf to certain sounds, but become anxious around other sounds, such as that of a vacuum cleaner or electric mixer. In many autistic children, the sense of touch, taste, hearing, sight, or smell seems to be out of focus or distorted. Toe walking is a common behavior in autistic children (Weber, 1978) and seems to be associated with tactile perception. Toilet training is often difficult to accomplish, and mothers often report difficulties with elimination beginning in infancy. Peculiar food preferences and unusual sleep patterns are common among autistic children (Paluszny, 1979). Many of these disturbances improve with age, though the difficulties never completely disappear (Ando, Yoshimura, & Wakabayash, 1980).

Perceptual disturbances have been related to the faulty modulation of sensory input; in other words, the regulators of sensory stimuli reaching the brain do not work properly. There may be too little or too much information or exaggerated responses to incoming information, all alternating within the same child (Ornitz, 1978; Ornitz & Ritvo, 1976).

The notion that autistic children have unimpaired intellectual functioning has been laid to rest. Only 20 percent of autistic children have normal or above normal intelligence (Rutter, 1978a); the remaining 80 percent function in the retarded or severely retarded range. Autism and mental retardation are not mutually exclusive (Carr, 1976). Severely autistic individuals may have normal or above normal intelligence; however, autistic children with low I.Q. scores are just as retarded as anyone else with a low I.Q. score (Rutter, 1978a). Kanner considered autism to be a specific disease syndrome rather than a syndrome on a continuum of certain developmental disabilities (Schopler, Reichler, DeVellis, & Daly, 1980). However, studies have shown that one-third to one-half of autistic children have associated central nervous system dysfunction (L. Wing, 1979), coupled with a range of retardation (Carr, 1976) and perceptual disorders (Rutter, 1978a). Therefore, the view that autism consists of a range of disabilities is increasingly more acceptable. Even among those children who are severely retarded, there may be some who have a few specific skills that they could perform at or near their chronological age level (Carr, 1976; M.K. DeMyer, Barton, W.E. DeMyer, Norton, Allen, & Steele, 1973).

The cognitive and perceptual deficits of autistic children have been a puzzle to educators and therapists since the syndrome was first described. As Eisenberg (1956) has noted, "severely autistic children exhibit a preoccupation with the sensory impressions stemming from the world about them, but seem unable to organize perceptions into functional patterns" (p. 611). Indeed, autistic children seem to have no organized system for thinking about past events, for interpreting the present, and for planning for the future (Hermelin, 1971). Autistic persons seem unable to think in abstract terms. Because of this inability to process incoming information and relate it to old information, things appear to happen in a haphazard and random way. The only help is to provide structure and organization from the outside (L. Wing, 1979).

The problems of severely retarded autistic children are, of course, more difficult to deal with. Self-injury, stereotypic movements, extreme self-stimulation, lack of responsiveness, and profound inability to communicate are common, as are physical disabilities. These children have great difficulty in learning new skills, and they are often subject to extremes of mood fluctuation (Carr, 1976).

INCIDENCE AND PROGNOSIS

The incidence of autism varies, according to the method used in sampling the population and the criteria used for diagnosis. The National Society for Children and Adults with Autism (1980) reports that 5 out of every 10,000 births will produce an autistic child. Other studies place the incidence at 4 or 5 in every 10,000 (L. Wing, 1972) and 2 to 4 in 10,000 cases (American Psychiatric Association, 1980). These statistics suggest that autism is a rare disorder; however, autism occurs as often as total deafness in childhood and more often than total blindness (L. Wing, 1972).

Autism occurs in families throughout the world, in all racial, ethnic, and social backgrounds. While it seems that no group is excluded from the disorder, studies have shown that it affects more boys than girls, in a ratio of about four to one (Rutter, 1978a; L. Wing, 1972). However, girls with autism are generally more severely affected than boys (Tsai, Stewart, & August, 1981).

About one-third of all autistic children have some other handicap affecting brain or central nervous system function (L. Wing, 1972). Such conditions include spasticity, epilepsy, hydrocephalitis, and so on (Ornitz & Ritvo, 1976).

The prognosis for autistic individuals is, at present, not bright. Recent studies indicate that the two most valuable predictors of outcome are intellectual functioning and language (Harper & Williams, 1975; Rimland, 1964). In a study by M.K. DeMyer et al. (1973), it was reported that the children who were functioning at normal or near normal levels were those who had communicative speech by age five. Lotter (1974) reported that, in a follow-up study of 32 autistic children, speech and I.Q. together were the critical indicators of outcome.

In another study (S.C. Res & Taylor, 1975), a list of 23 items that were correlated with successful prognosis for autistic children indicated that 100 percent of those children who had a successful outcome had an I.Q. above 70, and 75 percent of those who had a successful outcome made the greatest amount of behavioral change during their first month of treatment. Of those who made a successful adjustment, 65 percent displayed some appropriate use of toys, and 60 percent had some communicative language at the beginning of treatment.

In a classic follow-up study of 80 autistic children, Eisenberg (1956) noted that failure to develop speech—or having lost speech—was equal to a poor prognosis. Prognosis, then, according to Eisenberg, was based on the presence of "useful" speech by age five. In this study, about 50 percent of those children who had useful speech by age five were able to make a good social adjustment. All of the cases who had no speech made a poor adjustment.

While Eisenberg isolated speech as a predictor of outcome, other authors found that I.Q. is the best predictor. Rutter (1978a) indicated that the I.Q. score is a reasonable predictor of later educational progress. The American Psychiatric Association (1980) noted that those factors most closely related to long-term progress are I.Q. and the development of language skills. Sixty to seventy-five percent of autistic children have poor or very poor prognoses (M.K. DeMyer et al., 1973). According to the American Psychiatric Association (1980), one out of six will make an adequate social adjustment and will be able to do some kind of work; one out of six will make a fair adjustment; and the remaining two-thirds will continue to be handicapped for the rest of their lives.

CAUSAL FACTORS

Though theories abound, no single cause of the syndrome of autism has been isolated. Researchers have studied the relationship between autism and viruses (Stubbs, Crawford, Burger, & Vandenbark, 1977; Stubbs & Magenis, 1980); but, while these theories are interesting, they are as yet inconclusive. Stubbs (1978) found a case of autism occurring in conjunction with cytomegalovirus (CMV). Other evidence to support the viral impact theory is reported by Stubbs et al. (1977) and Torrey (1980). In a study of 243 children with congenital rubella, Chess (1977) found that there was a high rate of autism among the subjects. Though there seems to be a correlation between viral impact and some subgroups of autistic individuals, the presence of a virus does not account for all cases of autism.

A second theory is that the syndrome of autism is caused by a metabolic disorder; that is, the body processes certain chemicals erroneously or fails to process certain substances needed for brain functions to work properly (Coleman, 1973; Rimland, 1976; Shearer, Larsen, Neuschwander, & Gedney, 1982). A number of studies have shown that there may be some validity to this theory:

- Yuwiler, Geller, and Ritvo (1976) sampled over 70 subjects and found somewhat higher levels of serotonin in blood platelets of autistics. They noted, however, that the meaning of these results was uncertain. They did not conclude that their findings indicated a causal relationship between serotonin levels in the brain and autism, but they did note that the results deserved further investigation.
- In a study of the effects of large doses of vitamin B-15, Rimland (1979) found that improved speech and awareness resulted from this type of therapy for many of the autistic subjects.
- Coleman (1980) found that more parents of autistic children had problems with hyperthyroidism in the preconception period. The number of such parents differed substantially from that in the control group. She also found that serotonin, a chemical neurotransmitter necessary for synaptic transmission, tended to be elevated in the majority of autistic children studied. However, in ten percent of the autistic population studied, serotonin levels were found to be very low. For those ten percent, it was found that vitamin B-6 and magnesium improved sleeping and attention span.
- LeLord, Muh, Barthelemy, Martineau, Garreau, and Callaway (1981) administered large doses of vitamin B-6 and magnesium to 44 autistic children and found clinical improvement in 15 of the subjects. The improvements were described as increased alertness, reduction in emotional outbursts, reduced negativism, reduced self-mutilation, and reduction of stereotypic behavior. The researchers noted that they were unable to isolate clinical indicators of candidates who would be more likely to improve with such treatment. However, those who did show improvement seemed to be male, younger, retarded in growth, and to have had an earlier onset of the disorder.

Contradictory findings related to the metabolic dysfunction in autism have also been reported (Sverd, Kupietz, Winsberg, Hurwic, & Becker, 1978). Jackson and Garrod (1978) measured plasma zinc, copper, and amino acid levels in autistic children, and found the levels to be within normal limits. Young, Kyprie, Ross, and Cohen (1980) reported that, in a study of serum dopamine-beta-hydroxylase in 44 autistic children, the levels did not differ significantly from those in the general population. D. J. Cohen, Young, Lowe, and Harcherik (1980) studied thyroid functioning in 58 autistics. They found no differences between autistics and normals.

Rodnight (1978) noted that, in any normal population, individual biochemical differences play some part in influencing behavior patterns. Therefore, until more sophisticated tools for studying brain chemicals and the effect of metabolic functioning on behavior are found, research into this area will remain tentative. Thus, while the above studies are promising, they are by no means conclusive. Though they show a relationship between the abnormal presence or absence of substances needed for normal functioning, they provide us with little empirical information regarding behavioral effects.

Other researchers are investigating the relationship between autism and structural brain damage. Abnormalities of the temporal lobe (DeLong, 1978) and the limbic system (Goldman, 1979; Torrey, 1980), abnormal EEG (M.K. DeMyer, 1979; Torrey, 1980), and minor physical anomalies (Links, 1980; Links, Stockwell, Abichandani, & Simeon, 1980) all indicate a possible relationship with autistic behaviors. Walker (1977) suggests that the minor physical anomalies exhibited by many autistic children is evidence for concluding that congenital factors are at least associated with the presence of autism.

Weir and Salisbury (1980) support the hypothesis that autistic symptoms may occur as a result of brain damage at or before birth. In a case study of a child who suffered prolonged unconsciousness, they reported the appearance of severe eye-to-eye gaze avoidance, sensory inattention, and other behavioral symptoms of autism. These symptoms disappeared, however, after a few months.

Perhaps one of the most interesting and most recent areas of study in relation to autism is that of the brain stem. Student and Sohmer (1978), Rosenblum, Arick, Krug, Stubbs, Young, and Pelson (1980), and Tanguay and Edwards (1982) reported that auditory brain-stem-evoked responses indicated organic brain stem lesions in autistic children. Other studies using electrophysicological measures of brain function have shown similar results (Etemad, Szurek, Yeager, & Schulkin, 1973; Hauser, DeLong, & Rosman, 1975).

Several studies have focused on the function of various areas of the brain and cortical substructures that when damaged, may cause various autistic symptoms (Goldman, 1979; Ornitz, 1974; Ornitz, Tanguay, Lee, Ritvo, Silvertsen, & Wilson, 1972; Small, 1971; Towbin, 1978; Tsai et al., 1981). One such area is a group of cortical substructures generally known as the limbic system. For years, researchers believed that the limbic system primarily controlled or regulated emotional states. More recently, it has been suggested that the limbic system plays a part in the regulation of social and communicative responses, particularly the prelinguistic, extralinguistic, and nonverbal aspects of human behavior (Berry, 1980; DeLong, 1978). Lamendella (1977) speculates that, in view of the functions attributed to the limbic system, these substructures may be implicated in the syndrome of autism. Though Lamendella's hypothesis is speculative and theoretical, it is worth mentioning, since research into this area is still new.

Chromosomal or genetic factors are also believed to be suspect in the etiology of autism, though not all autistic persons are autistic due to genetic inheritance or chromosomal disorders (Tsai et al., 1981). Coleman (1980) has suggested that there may be a genetic predisposition that causes a subgroup of the autistic population to be vulnerable to the disorder. Studies of twins and autistic siblings are beginning to shed some light on the theory of genetic predisposition (Rutter & Lockyer, 1967; Sloan, 1978). However, the studies have thus far failed to show conclusively chromosomal abnormalities in any subgroup of autistic children (Spence, 1976).

It is unlikely that there is one single factor that causes autism (L. Wing, 1976). Coleman (1980) suggests that there are probably many subgroups of the disorder and that each may have its own unique causal factor.

It should be evident from the foregoing discussion that autism is, as yet, not understood, either in terms of the cause or causes, or in terms of prevention and cure. What *is* known is that the terribly incapacitating consequences of the disorder are the result of some type of brain or central nervous system malfunction. At present, treatment is based on symptoms rather than the cause (Fish, 1976b). While professionals await medical science's answers, our best treatment consists of modifying the disturbances of behavior that are manifestations of underlying physiological disorders.

DIAGNOSIS

Autism is not always easy to diagnose, given the various opinions regarding the criteria for autism. Autism may occur in conjunction with mental retardation or a variety of other handicapping conditions. The question that inevitably arises is, What is the purpose of diagnosis?

The need for assigning a "label" to an individual depends upon the intended use of that label. That is, a diagnosis may be given for any number of reasons. For clinical and research purposes, the diagnosis may be reserved for those individuals who show, prior to 36 months of age, irregularities of development and disturbances of the modulation of sensory input, relatedness, and language (Ornitz & Ritvo, 1976). For public school placement and intervention, a broader diagnostic category may be desirable (L. Wing, 1976). Although the necessity for a complete medical and neurological evaluation may be strongly recommended (Ornitz & Ritvo, 1976), the actual medical diagnosis may do little to help the teacher or clinician in developing intervention procedures to help autistic children.

Persons with autism are diagnosed as such because they demonstrate certain behaviors that cluster together to form a pattern. The various component behaviors—such as deviant language, social relatedness, perception, cognition, and so on—can be described by any number of formal or informal tests or checklists. However, there is no physical or psychological measurement that will confirm the diagnosis of autism. Autism is defined by a pattern of behaviors (Marcus, 1978). Generally, a medical diagnosis is based on the criteria described in the first section of this chapter. Obviously, these criteria do not always agree, and diagnoses may differ, depending upon the biases of the professionals who are performing the diagnosing.

Diagnosis becomes important when certain educational procedures or techniques are required. For example, Arick and Krug (1978) found that autistic students require four times more trials to learn the first step of a sequencing task than they do for the remaining steps. Thus, the autistic individual presents a significant learning-to-learn curve. Autistic children require a great deal of effort and expert instruction in order for improvement to occur. In many cases, instruction is effective only in a highly structured teaching environment that provides a high teacher/low student ratio (Krug, Arick, & Almond, 1980). Diagnosis, then, is important primarily to the professional working with autistic individuals.

Although selection for training should be based on behaviors rather than on the "label" (O'Dell, Blackwell, Larcen, & Hogaw, 1977), there are some diagnostic tools that help to provide a means of differentiating autism from other disorders. Several of these diagnostic tools are described below. Professionals who use these tools must keep in mind that they are measures of behavior and, as such, they have their limitations. They should be used as aids in designing educational or therapeutic programs; they should not be considered definitive diagnostic instruments in themselves.

Diagnostic Criteria

For many years, professionals have relied upon various criteria in giving a diagnosis of autism (American Psychiatric Association, 1980; Creak, 1961; Kanner, 1943; National Society for Children and Adults with Autism, 1980; Rimland, 1964). In an effort to define autism objectively, checklists have been developed (Freeman, Schroth, Ritvo, Guthrie, & Wake, 1980; Rimland, 1964, 1971; Schopler, et al., 1980) the administration and interpretation of which is sometimes dubious, at best (Metcalf, 1973). The essential question for any professional involved in the diagnosis of a handicapped child is, What purpose will the diagnosis serve?

In the world of medicine, it is generally accepted that the diagnosis of a particular disease or disorder leads to the prescription for the cure or, at least, to alleviation of the symptoms. The label (naming the disorder) becomes important, then, only in proportion to the amount of remedial information it provides or implies.

For example, a diagnosis of otitis media (ear infection) tells the physician that certain remedial procedures must be followed, that is, specific medication must be provided, in order to prevent the disease from causing permanent hearing loss to the affected individual. In cases of specific diseases and their known remedies, diagnostic labels are critical. Such is not the case, however, with autism. There is still much confusion over the term, as well as over the behaviors that constitute the syndrome. Autism is a description of symptoms rather than a diagnostic entity. The label *autism* does not imply consequent medical (or any other) treatment for the remediation of a disease. Therefore, any assessment procedure that sets out to define an individual as autistic (as opposed to retarded, psychotic, and so forth) must answer the question, To what purpose?

Diagnostic Tools

There is no point in describing an individual as autistic if a prescription for remedy is not, at least, implicit. Essentially, until medical science finds a remedy for the underlying causes of autism, the course of treatment continues to focus on behavioral symptoms. The diagnostic tool that is most valuable to the educator or clinician is one that describes an individual's limitations in all areas of functioning and draws attention to a process for remediation (Newsom & Rincover, 1981). Two such diagnostic instruments are described below. They are included here because of their value as "prescriptive" tests of behaviors associated with autism.

Individualized Assessment and Treatment for Autistic and
　　Developmentally Disabled Children: The Psychoeducational
　　Profile

The Psychoeducational Profile (PEP) (Schopler & Reichler, 1979) is based on a developmental approach to the assessment of autistic children with related developmental disabilities. As an assessment tool, it provides information on developmental functioning in the areas of imitation, perception, fine and gross motor skills, eye-hand integration, cognitive performance, and cognitive verbal skills. As a diagnostic tool, the PEP identifies the degree of disorganized and disturbed behaviors present in a child, as well as the specific areas in which these behaviors are found.

There are 95 items in the developmental function areas. The imitation scale consists of 10 items that assess the child's ability to imitate both verbally and motorically, for example, to imitate gross body movements, to tap a bell twice after a demonstration, and to imitate sounds such as /m/.

The perception scale consists of 11 items designed to evaluate functioning in the areas of visual and auditory perception. For example, scale items test the ability to find an object hidden under a cup after the cup has been rotated with another, to follow visually the movement of bubbles, and to orient to the sound of a whistle.

The fine motor and gross motor scales are composed of 10 items and 11 items, respectively. Fine motor items test such abilities as opening a lid on a jar, cutting with scissors, and stringing beads. The gross motor items test abilities like walking alone, climbing stairs, and balancing on one foot.

The eye-hand integration scale, comprised of 14 items, evaluates eye-hand coordination and fine motor skills. Scale items test such abilities as scribbling on paper, coloring on lines, copying a circle and square, and stacking blocks.

The cognitive performance and cognitive verbal scales are designed to assess cognition. They require some language competence. The cognitive performance scale consists of 20 items testing performance tasks that do not require a direct verbal response. However, some understanding of language is required. The cognitive verbal scale contains 19 items that require a verbal response. Item tasks include counting aloud, solving simple arithmetic problems, sorting cards into sets by color and form, and pointing to and naming objects in a picture book.

The second part of the PEP is the pathology scale. The 44 items in this scale are designed to identify pathological or psychotic behaviors. The specific subunits of (1) affect; (2) relating, cooperating, and human interest; (3) play and interest in materials; (4) sensory modes; and (5) language are useful in defining the degree and type of structure needed by the child. Items in the pathology scale test such things as maintaining eye contact, exploring test materials appropriately, showing normal interest in smells, using words in an appropriate manner, and using unstructured time.

Expanded use of the test gives the evaluator information about the child's frustration tolerance and social understanding, and also provides an environment for teaching new skills. The total time required to administer and score the 139 items on the PEP is between 45 and 75 minutes, with an average testing time of one hour.

The PEP is designed to identify uneven and idiosyncratic learning patterns. It is most appropriately used with children functioning at a preschool age level who are in the chronological age range of 1 to 12 years. Developmental age norms are provided for all areas of function, so that the child's performance in each function area and overall level of performance can be compared with profiles of normal children at the same age levels. The total PEP score correlates highly with several intelligence tests; however, the PEP is designed primarily for planning instructional programs rather than for arriving at a summary or I.Q. score. Its authors suggest that, with children who have highly uneven patterns of abilities, it is more important to know the relative strengths and weaknesses in the various developmental areas than it is to obtain an I.Q. score.

The PEP is easily administered and scored, and it possesses several qualities not generally found in standardized assessment tools. First, successful performance on most items is not dependent upon the child's language skills. Second, the administration of the test permits observation and flexibility in dealing with the child's behavioral limitations. There are no timed items; and the scoring system is unique in the sense that, in addition to a "pass" or "fail" score, it may be shown that the skill is "emerging." Emerging indicates that the child has some knowledge of what is required to complete a task, but does not have the full understanding or ability to complete the task successfully. This unique category is important for the development of individual learning programs.

The scores on the PEP are designed to be translated into teaching strategies or programs for individual children. To help accomplish this goal, Volume II of the Individualized Assessment for Autistic and Developmentally Disabled Children was developed (Schopler, Reichler, & Lansing, 1980). This volume presents teaching hierarchies and teaching goals and expectations that combine the developmental perspective with behavioral techniques. In addition, a model for parent and professional involvement is presented.

The Autism Screening Instrument for Educational Planning

The Autism Screening Instrument for Educational Planning (ASIEP) (Krug et al., 1980) was designed to facilitate screening of autistic children for placement and educational intervention. The instrument consists of five subcomponents, each of which can also be used alone to assess a particular area. The "autism screening checklist," a checklist of 47 nonadaptive behaviors, provides a profile of the individual compared to other populations with handicapping conditions. This checklist of behavioral characteristics presents a profile that differentiates individuals who have been diagnosed autistic from all others with handicapping conditions. The "sample of vocal behavior" analyzes repetitiveness, noncommunication, intelligibility, and babbling. The profile obtained using these measures provides information that aids in differential diagnosis.

The "interaction assessment" examines the individual's ability to relate. This subtest uses direct observation of the individual's responses to an adult in a play setting and gives a summary profile chart that compares the individual's performance with a standardized sample.

The "educational assessment" subtest provides guidelines for beginning work with the autistic individual. This subtest examines (1) in-seat activity, to see if the individual will stay in a seat and cooperate; (2) receptive language, to measure understanding and response to auditory and verbal stimuli; (3) expressive language to assess responses (verbal, sign, or gestural) to questions about the immediate environment; (4) body concept, to evaluate motor skills and body identification knowledge; and (5) speech imitation, to assess the ability to articulate a variety of vocalizations.

The "prognosis of learning rate" analyzes the autistic child's learning rates and stimulus overselectivity compared to other diagnostic groups (see the discussion of stimulus overselectivity in Chapter 2). This subtest assesses educational learning potential by means of a simple two-step, black/white sequencing task.

For each component of the ASIEP, comparative profiles from autistic and nonautistic, severely retarded children are provided.

The ASIEP is designed to be a tool for educators in providing appropriate services for autistic students and for facilitating placement of autistic children into individual instructional settings with reduced student-teacher ratios. The scores on the various subtests indicate the degree to which an individual's deficits obstruct learning and the degree to which a highly specialized, structured educational environment must be provided.

A manual, *Autistic and Severely Handicapped in the Classroom: Assessment, Behavior Management, and Communication Training* (Krug, Rosenblum, Almond, & Arick, 1981), supplements the ASIEP by providing a systematic procedure for instructing autistic children in the classroom. The manual provides an overview of a communication-based curriculum and specific strategies for teaching communication, for assessing severely developmentally delayed individuals, and for implementing behavior management techniques.

SUMMARY

The syndrome of autism is a seriously incapacitating disorder. Autistic individuals differ from each other, just as nonautistic individuals differ from each other. Yet, there are some distinguishing characteristics that all autistic individuals share. Autism is a behavioral syndrome and, as such, may be described by listing a set of behaviors that distinguish autistic persons from individuals with other kinds of disorders. The behaviors that describe autism are (1) onset of the disorder before the age of 30 months, (2) impaired social relationships, (3) failure to develop communication skills, and (4) abnormal responses to the environment. Autism may occur in conjunction with mental retardation or a variety of other handicaps, or it may occur alone. The intellectual capabilities of autistic individuals vary widely, with the majority functioning in the retarded range.

It is estimated that 5 out of every 10,000 individuals are autistic. Males are affected four times more often than females. Prognosis for the child affected with autism is not good, although language development and intelligence have been shown to make a difference in outcome. Physiological causes have been suggested; however, no single cause for the syndrome has, as yet, been identified. Most likely, there are numerous subgroups of the disorder, each possessing its own etiology.

The purpose of diagnosis is to provide evidence for educational placement and to provide information for planning intervention. Two diagnostic instruments used for designing educational and therapeutic programs are the Individualized Assessment and Treatment for Autistic and Developmentally Disabled Children: The Psychoeducational Profile (PEP) and the Autism Screening Instrument for Educational Planning (ASIEP). These assessment instruments are prescriptive; that is, they assess learning deficits and prescribe areas for individualized instructional programming.

Chapter 2

Communicative Behavior of Autistic Children

One of the most interesting and baffling symptoms of autism is the unusual quality of language and communicative behavior. Kanner (1943) was fascinated with the type of language performance exhibited by his original autistic patients. He described their language as echolalic, literal, metaphorical, and seemingly irrelevant or noncommunicative. However, in his descriptive essay on the autistic's use of language, Kanner (1946) took great pains to explain how seemingly irrelevant or metaphorical utterances could be traced to their original source. In so doing, he found that the autistic children he observed were substituting or transferring meanings from the original source and applying them in new situations. The metaphorical expressions, according to Kanner, had a private, original source for meaning, known only to the child, unless the source could be traced. He suggested that this private use of language was unique to the autistic syndrome and that it stemmed primarily from the inability to use language in a socially communicative fashion.

The mutism that Kanner observed in eight of his patients (Kanner, 1946) was characterized by a consistent lack of speech, interrupted only rarely by whole sentences in emergency situations.

Kanner's descriptions of autistic children would lead one to assume that there are two types of language behavior exhibited by autistics. One type is the mute individual, who "chooses" not to speak, except on rare occasions; on such occasions the speech is apparently normal. The second type is the verbal autistic person, whose speech and language behavior is noncommunicative, literal, echolalic, and somehow suggestive of psychopathology. The presumed psychopathology inferred from deviant autistic speech was a predominant issue in the treatment of autistic children for many years (Creak, 1972).

Studies have attempted to show that mothers of autistic children were different from mothers of normal children in their speech and conversation with their children (W. Goldfarb, Yadkovitz, & N. Goldfarb, 1973). Professionals have attempted to explain the deviant use of pronouns and other relational concepts as evidence of an inability to perceive the self as an entity (Despert, 1968). Subsequent studies have shown, however, that the deviant language of autistic individuals is indicative neither of the presence of psychiatric disorder nor of mothers with defective communication or conversational skills (Bartak & Rutter, 1974; Cantwell, L. Baker, & Rutter, 1977).

In the four decades since Kanner first described the syndrome, the various disciplines that deal with autistic children have come a long way in the theory and practice of treating such children. Yet, most professionals continue to rely, in almost slavish fashion, on the early, rather meager descriptions provided by Kanner.

Because of the narrowness of the diagnostic criteria, early descriptions of the language of autistic children were limited to the language behavior of those autistic children who possessed, as Kanner described it, good cognitive abilities (Kanner, 1943). Except for a few recent works (Fay & Schuler, 1980; Needleman, Ritvo, & Freeman, 1980), relevant studies have failed to analyze fully the linguistic and communicative behavior of autistic children. More particularly, they have failed to describe and analyze the communicative behavior of the nonverbal, or mute, autistic child.

Professionals now recognize that a very limited number of autistic individuals possess normal or above normal intellectual potential. Autistic children do not possess cognitive qualities that are mysteriously "locked up." J.K. Wing (1976) effectively summed up this critical realization:

> Autistic children do have a fascination which lies partly in the feeling that somewhere there must be a key which will unlock hidden treasure. The skilled searcher will indeed find treasure . . . but the currency will be everyday and human, not fairy gold. In return for our attention, these children may give us the key to human language, which is the key to humanity itself. (p. 14)

The task of this chapter, therefore, is to present a description of the communicative and linguistic behavior of those autistic children who do speak and who possess some form of language competence, and then to focus on the communicative behavior and interrelated aspects of cognition, perception, and social competence of the nonverbal autistic child.

CHARACTERISTICS OF THE VERBAL AUTISTIC CHILD

The question of whether or not the autistic's language production differs substantially from that of other types of language disorders has been the focus of some attention (Menyuk, 1978; Pierce & Bartolucci, 1977; Tager-Flusberg, 1981). Needleman et al. (1980) compared the verbal performance of 33 autistic children with the verbal performance of mentally retarded and other language-delayed subjects. The characteristics that were found to set autistic verbal behavior apart from other types of language disorders were imprecise articulation, echolalia, perseveration on question type, atypical intonation, atypical stress, and stereotypic expressions. Two-thirds of the autistic children studied exhibited three or more of these characteristics. The mentally retarded subjects, in contrast, demonstrated uniform expressive and receptive language levels, generalized compre-hension, and the presence of an identifiable expressive developmental level. The language behavior of the autistic child is specific and different from that of the mentally retarded child.

Autistic children's communicative behavior is also different from such behavior in other types of disorders. Often, parents of young autistic children first seek professional help because they suspect that their non-speaking child may be deaf. However, unlike the autistic child who is broadly unresponsive, the deaf child is unresponsive only to sounds (Pal-uszny, 1979). Gross deficits in speech often present problems for the diagnostician (L. Baker, Cantwell, Rutter, & Bartak, 1976). The commu-nicative behavior of the autistic child can be contrasted with the commu-nication pattern of the aphasic individual. In contrast to autistic speech, which is often monotonic, aphasic speech has normal pitch, stress, and intonation. Echolalia is more frequent in autistics; and, when it is present in aphasics, it is generally used in appropriate contexts. Aphasics use gestures to facilitate communication, whereas autistics do not. The aphasic has creative and imaginative play, suggestive of an inner language and intact skills for organizing and interpreting the environment. Aphasics are more likely to be spontaneous in their attempts to use speech and less likely to be echolalic and stereotypic (B.L. Baker, Brightman, Heifetz, & Murphy, 1976). Autistic individuals are more prone than aphasics to avoid eye contact, lack friends, have limited group play skills, involve them-selves in ritualistic behaviors, and show excessive sensitivity to sounds (Rutter, 1978b).

Echolalia

Echolalia is one of the most characteristic behaviors observed in the autistic child (Needleman et al., 1980). Echolalia is defined as the inappro-priate repetition of words, phrases, or sentences previously spoken by others (W. Goldfarb, N. Goldfarb, Braunstein, & Scholl, 1972; Schuler, 1979). The echolalic behavior of autistic children has been studied at length, and three types of echolalia have emerged (Baltaxe & Simmons, 1975; Fay & Schuler, 1980; Schuler, 1979).

1. *Immediate echolalia* is the verbatim repetition of utterances following their occurrence. Immediate echolalia may involve the repetition of the whole or part of the utterance. For example, when asked, "Do you want some juice?" five-year-old Sally replies, "Some juice?" Immediate repetition of the last word or words of questions put to her is a consistent verbal behavior for Sally. The echoed words precisely duplicate the pitch, stress, intonation, and articulation patterns of the speaker.

2. *Delayed echolalia* involves the literal repetition of an utterance sometime after the original utterance. Repetition of commercials, lines from familiar songs, or parts of television programs are typical examples of delayed echolalia. Autistic children have been known to flawlessly repeat zip codes or addresses that they have heard on radio or television. A typical example is the child who shouted, "Write Washington D.C. 20202," whenever he saw a photograph of a building that resembled the colonnaded, stone government buildings in Washington, D.C.

3. *Mitigated echolalia* involves the repetition of utterances that deviate slightly from the original. Variations of the original are accomplished by deletions, additions, or intonation changes (Schuler, 1979). It is sometimes difficult to recognize mitigated echolalia for what it is, since the repetition is not exact, nor does the repeated utterance have to occur immediately following the original utterance. The following exchange between an autistic adolescent and his therapist may serve to illustrate the phenomenon:

> *Therapist:* David, if you want to earn points, you have to first clear off the table.
> *David:* Yes, Debbie. If you want to earn points, you have to clear off the table, don't I, Debbie?

Another example of mitigated echolalia is the child who, after having been told once by her mother, "Now, don't you wet the bed tonight, Janie," consistently repeats, "Now, don't you wet the bed tonight, Anne (mother's name)," every night as she climbs into bed.

Fay and Schuler (1980) have suggested that, while mitigated echolalia is not a useful communication device for the autistic individual, it demonstrates that language does intervene. Often, as in the examples above, proper names or personal pronouns are omitted or exchanged. The result is linguistic chaos. Nevertheless, the utterance may reflect the partial ability or emerging potential to comprehend the relationships expressed in syntactic or structural rules for language usage.

Fay and Schuler (1980) also suggest that immediate echolalia indicates that the message has failed to register and that the echoed response is merely "triggered" by stimuli extrinsic to the child. Delayed echolalia, on the other hand, may be triggered by an appropriate similar context and may contain communicative intent. Metaphoric speech, in which private meaning is attached or transferred to subsequent events, is likely to be nothing more than delayed (and sometimes mitigated) echolalia (Kanner, 1946).

The echolalic response triggered by some event seems to have some internal significance for the child, expressed in the form of the literal repetition of a phrase or sentence (Fay & Schuler, 1980). Consider, for example, the child whose verbal repertoire consists primarily of the delayed or mitigated repetition of television commercials and radio jingles. The echolalic responses produced by this child, however, are evidently quite appropriately placed in social contexts. For example, the child pauses between bites of a huge piece of delicious chocolate cake and exclaims, "Mmm! Tastes good, Mom! Moist and rich. Betty Crocker." The television devotee will immediately recognize the mitigated, echoed commercial for Betty Crocker cake mixes. This shared information is restricted to a very limited audience. It is restrictive in the sense that only those who recall the commercial can make sense out of the autistic child's words. The obvious question here is, Does this child *intend* to communicate something to someone, or is the response a purely behavioral one, stimulated or triggered by the presence of the chocolate cake? Is the verbal utterance a spontaneous attempt to socialize, even though the form is stereotypic, or is the verbal utterance a simple behavioral reflex or verbal self-stimulation?

Echolalia seems to have a functional purpose in the normal developmental process, in as much as it is a temporary phenomenon in a continuum of behavioral change, from the more automatic or mechanical to the purposeful use of speech (Fay & Schuler, 1980). The imitative behavior of the normally developing child is rarely mere mimicry (the meaningless repetition of a behavior). Normal echolalic behavior, which disappears by the end of the second year of life, seems to serve as a means of testing the structure of language and of evaluating one's own language as it stacks up against other language users in the environment (Menyuk, 1978). It has been suggested that echolalic autistic children do not "pass through" this imitative stage, as normal children do. Rather, they seem to develop a form of vocal repetition that becomes a form of self-stimulation (Lovaas, 1968).

In contrast to this point of view, others have suggested that echolalic behavior may represent the autistic child's attempt to bridge the communication gap (Baltaxe & Simmons, 1977). Prizant and Duchan (1981) suggest that immediate echolalia in autistic individuals may be nonfunctional, but alternatively, it may perform one or more of the following functions: turn-taking, declaration, rehearsal, self-regulation, yes-answer, or request.

Careful observation of the concrete repetition of verbal events may provide the professional with clues about the way autistic children view the world (Paluszny, 1979). The echolalic behavior of the verbal autistic child may reflect a concrete, literal interpretation of events; it may also indicate an inability to process or use linguistic information appropriately. Paccia and Curcio (1982) analyzed autistic children's responses to sentence completion tasks, "wh" questions, and "yes/no" questions. They found that echolalia occurred significantly more often following a yes/no question. They concluded that there could be a relationship between autistic echolalia and the difficulty of the linguistic structure; that is, echolalia is more likely to occur following uncomprehended questions. The difficulty with the yes/no dichotomy, like the failure to appreciate relational contrasts evidenced by the familiar pronominal reversal (using "you" for "I"), reflects the autistic child's concrete and literal use of speech. The inability to formulate general principles, to draw inferences, or to perceive subtly transmitted rules is manifest in the autistic speaker's failure to comprehend or evolve word definitions, similarities, differences, common denominators, logical analogies, opposites, metaphors, and causality (Baltaxe & Simmons, 1975).

Other Deviant Communicative Behaviors

The deviant use of personal pronouns stems from the inability to understand the morphological function of abstract relationships, and time-related concepts (Bartolucci & Albers, 1974). The personal pronouns I and you are repeated as heard. Bartak and Rutter (1974) have demonstrated that, if the position of personal pronouns within a sentence is controlled, the autistic child does not avoid the use of "I" (as was once believed), but repeats it as heard. Thus, the child who echoes, "Do *you* want some juice?" will just as likely echo, "*I* want some juice."

The difficulty in responding to yes/no questions has already been mentioned. Rimland (1964) noted that asking or answering questions poses a particular problem for autistic children. He also noted that "No!" is frequently indicated by grunting or emphatically waving the arms. Judging from the suggestions made by Baltaxe and Simmons (1975) and Rimland (1964), it would seem that autistic children answer "yes" by echoing the question and answer "no" by grunting or emphatically waving the arms. The logical conclusion might be that the meaning of the question is understood, but the appropriate vehicle (the linguistic rule) is not available to the child. However, it has been demonstrated that autistic children can be taught to answer questions appropriately (Freeman, Ritvo, & R. Miller, 1975).

It is curious that, while their linguistic development is poor, autistic children generally appear to develop normal phonological abilities (Hermelin, 1971). If the child develops speech, transient articulation disorders may be present, but these disappear with maturation. As a group, autistic children do not deviate significantly from the phonological developmental patterns of nonautistic children (Fay & Schuler, 1980; Menyuk, 1978). Bartolucci, Pierce, Streiner, and Eppel (1976) reported that verbal autistic children show a normal, yet slowed, development of sounds; and Needleman et al. (1980) demonstrated that only 5 out of 33 autistic subjects exhibited articulation disorders. There are, of course, some verbal autistic children whose phonological development is very deviant. In such cases, the articulation deficit may or may not be functionally related to linguistic errors.

The speech of autistic individuals has been characterized as "wooden" (Baltaxe & Simmons, 1975), empty, parrot-like, and monotone (Rimland, 1964). The voice quality of autistic speakers is often hoarse, harsh, or hypernasal. Distortions of pitch frequently involve consistent, high-pitched sound production. Whispering, muttering, occasional loud ejaculations, poor volume control, and guttural noises are common. Insufficient pitch changes, monotony, sing-song rhythm, and artificial (echolalic) stress contribute to the overall impression that the speech of the autistic individual is empty, devoid of social appropriateness, and noncommunicative.

Autistic children seem unable to use language to convey meaning to others (Cunningham & Dixon, 1961; Kanner, 1957). Every normal communicative act is made in a particular context and must be interpreted in the light of relevant information given in that context (Lyons, 1972). Language becomes communication when the components of language (syntax, semantics, and phonology) are used to convey an intended message to alter the behavior, attitudes, or beliefs of a hearer (Lucas, 1980). Even those autistic children who acquire language skills are limited in their ability to converse; they do not use language to share messages (Menyuk, 1978). Even though syntax, semantics, and phonology may be correct, the ability to use language as a social event, in context, remains a problem. Autistic individuals fail to acquire finesse in their interactions with others.

Repetitive questioning is a common device used by autistic persons to initiate and maintain conversations (Hurtig, Ensrud, & Tomblin, 1982). Autistic individuals lack the conversational management skills to maintain the conversation by listening and responding. They control the conversation by perseverating on the question form. Though they may genuinely seek an exchange of information, they may ask a string of apparently unrelated questions or repeat familiar commands without regard for the listener's interest. They may perseverate on the topic (Bernard-Opitz, 1982), resist turn-taking, fail to make conversational transitions with appropriate pauses, or fail to perceive the listener's reactions of uncertainty, disbelief, agreement, and so on, and to adjust their verbal message accordingly (Richer, 1978).

Very young normal children use spontaneous speech to orient and guide their own activities (Slobin, 1971). However, spontaneous speech is rarely present in the language behavior of the autistic child. Autistic children can be trained to use spoken words to label objects, actions, and wants, to answer simple questions, and to follow instructions, but they seem locked into a concrete world in which only one dimension can be responded to at a time (Churchill, 1978).

CHARACTERISTICS OF THE NONVERBAL AUTISTIC CHILD

Deviant Communication Development

It is estimated that nearly 50 percent of autistic individuals are mute (Rutter, 1978b). According to Fay and Schuler (1980), there are three levels of mutism. The first level is total muteness, that is, the absence of both communicative and noncommunicative vocalizations. The second level is functional mutism. Children who are functionally mute produce vocalizations that are used for self-stimulation or are involuntary emissions of noncommunicative sounds. The third level is semimutism. Semimute children show a limited repertoire of words and word approximations that are used in a functional way to express immediate desires or dislikes.

Since autistic children demonstrate uneven and deviant patterns of communicative development (Churchill, 1972; Rutter, 1978b), it may not be entirely appropriate to compare the language development of autistic individuals with that of a normal population (Prizant, 1982). However, an understanding of the early development of normal communication skills may be helpful in gaining some perspective regarding the nature of autistic communication.

Prior to the first year of life, normal infants respond to the mother's tone of voice. Before they begin to use speech, they respond by smiling, pointing, waving, and lifting their arms to be picked up (Menyuk, 1974). Normal infants of about nine months of age use their voices to attract attention, to express emotion, and to engage in social exchanges with familiar adults and use intonation to convey generalized meaning (McDonald, 1975b). As early as the first year of life, the normal child is able to use a variety of nonverbal means for communicative purposes (D.D. Bricker & Carlson, 1981). By the end of the first year, the child is capable of obeying simple verbal directions when accompanied by gestures. In the second year, the child displays a rich variety of articulate vocal play (babble) and begins to produce human speech sounds that are subsequently combined to form first words. The ability to comprehend adult linguistic forms may be present at these earliest one-word stages (Petretic & Tweney, 1977). In contrast, the autistic child fails to show the normal nonverbal prelinguistic skills mentioned above (M.K. DeMyer, 1979; Menyuk, 1978). Generally, the rich variety of babble and vocal experimentation is absent (Rutter, 1978a). Words may appear prior to 16–22 months, but disappear suddenly; delayed onset of speech is common (Fay & Schuler, 1980). Some researchers suggest that normal early language development is closely associated with the child's own actions and experiences (Dale, 1972; McDonald, 1975c; Rodgon, Jankowski, & Alenskas, 1977). The autistic child's failure to imitate (M.K. DeMyer et al., 1971) and to use objects appropriately in the environment (Rosenthal, Massie, & Wulff, 1980) may contribute to the already deficient prelinguistic communication skills. In the first year of life, the autistic child may not use sounds to indicate meaning or use the voice to attract attention or to show extremes of emotions, as normal infants do (Ricks & L. Wing, 1975). Many autistic children are expressionless (Rimland, 1964). Autistic children do not use gestures as substitutes for speech, but they may pull the adult by the hand to gain access to a desired object (Ricks & L. Wing, 1975). Even if speech develops, language is often reduced or telegraphic (Hermelin, 1971). Nonessential elements of grammar are frequently omitted, regardless of the complex language that the child may be able to use (Bartolucci et al., 1980).

Abnormal Paralinguistic Development

Social and communicative skills are so interrelated that they cannot be analyzed independently. Communication is a social act; participation in a communicative act with another individual requires certain prerequisite social/communicative skills that are evolved from species-specific rules for nonverbal behavior. Argyle (1972) has outlined the following nonverbal signals used by man:

- *Bodily contact.* The most common signals that involve bodily contact are those used to express greetings and farewell (for example, hand-shaking and waving "good-bye"). Other signals are hitting, pushing, stroking, hugging, and so on.
- *Proximity.* Cultural attitudes dictate how close people stand or sit to one another. Generally, people stand closer to people they like. Socially unskilled people are more distant. Changes in proximity indicate the desire to initiate or terminate an encounter.
- *Orientation.* The angle at which individuals sit or stand in relation to each other reflects the relationship. Sitting side by side indicates close friendship. Sitting or standing head-on indicates confrontation.
- *Appearance.* The clothes, hair, skin, and physique or bodily condition conveys a message about the individual's personality, mood, and social status.
- *Posture.* Ways of standing, sitting, and lying are used to convey interpersonal attitudes. Posture varies with emotional states.
- *Head nods.* The nod of the head is important in connection with speech. It is usually interpreted as permission to continue or as rein-forcement. Rapid head nods may indicate that the receiver of the message wants to speak.
- *Facial expressions.* Emotional expressions are conveyed by smiles, frowns, expansion of the pupils, and eye movements. The listener indicates puzzlement, surprise, disagreement, pleasure, and so on by small movements of the eyebrows and mouth. The speaker uses facial expressions to modify, emphasize, or punctuate what is being said. For example, facial expressions may indicate whether an utterance is intended to be funny, serious, important, or disgusting.
- *Gestures.* The hands are the most expressive parts of the body, but other body parts (feet, head) may be used to illustrate or support what is being said. Gestures may also be used to replace speech.
- *Looking.* During conversations, each participant looks intermittently at the other for periods of one to ten seconds, or for 25 to 75 percent of the time. Periods of mutual eye contact or gaze are shorter. Individuals look twice as much while listening as while talking.

The nonverbal, paralinguistic (Lyons, 1972) features of communication, according to Argyle (1972), play important roles in communicating inter-personal attitudes and establishing relationships. They are used to convey information and to support speech.

Autistic children fail to use these paralinguistic features of communication. If speech is present, gestures, eye movements, and facial expressions are not used in conjunction with what is being said in order to support or add information (Fay & Schuler, 1980). A study of 19 autistic subjects (Parry & Brandt, 1981) revealed that nonverbal autistic children used appropriate eye contact less frequently than did verbal autistics. Nonverbal autistics were less likely to differentiate familiar people from strangers; they initiated less contact with adults, produced more facial grimaces, and were more likely to engage in rigid and stereotypic object manipulation.

Cognitive Deficits

Unlike mentally retarded children, autistic children have a particular cognitive deficit that involves language and central coding processes related to sequencing and abstraction (Rutter, 1978a). The relationship of cognition to language competence is still under investigation (Rice, 1980); however, some inferences may be made in order to facilitate the understanding of communication development (Schlesinger, 1977).

In order to produce language the child must have something to talk about; the child must have inner language. The acquisition of inner language is dependent upon (1) the ability to acquire concepts and (2) the ability to code these into a symbol system for efficient recall (Paluszny, 1979).

Symbols represent ideas or concepts. The use of symbolization is a prelinguistic skill that makes it possible to conceive of alternatives to the here and now (Wolf & Gardner, 1981). Language is a symbolic system used for conveying ideas. Autistic persons seem to lack both the ability to interpret the symbols in their environment and to use the symbols to convey messages to others. The development of linguistic structures may reflect certain cognitive abilities, such as the ability to conceptualize experiences and to act upon the environment, which normally develops in the early months of life (Bowerman, 1976). The nonfunctional use of objects (Churchill, 1978), the failure to use toys for play (DesLauriers, 1978), the lack of gesture and imitative play (Menyuk, 1978), and the inability to consistently use pantomime (Curcio & Piserchia, 1978) are indicative of symbolic deficits. Cognitive symbolic deficits are found in the communicative behavior of autistic children (Kamhi, 1981). The capacity to produce and monitor the normal species-specific preverbal sounds is impaired; the desire to explore the environment, to form concepts, and to explain experiences is absent; and the ability to recognize that other human beings are of special interest and importance is lacking (L. Wing, 1981).

The distinction between noncommunicative and communicative (social) events can be made on the basis of "intent" (Kiernan, 1981). Communicative intent may be inferred when the behavior of one person deliberately affects the behavior of another person (Fay & Schuler, 1980). Intent is intimately related to social development, and is thought to be lacking in the autistic child (Paluszny, 1979).

Communicative intent is a difficult thing to judge. The issue is certainly more complex than it at first appears to be. Tantrums and self-destructive behavior are aversive to adults and could be used by autistic children to guarantee decreased social contact (Morrison, D. Miller, & Mejia, 1973). Yet, tantrums and other forms of inappropriate behavior may also be used by nonverbal children to gain access to adults and to express dislikes or desires. It is possible that autistic individuals do not deliberately avoid social contact, but lack the necessary skills for appropriate interaction (Howlin, 1978).

Other Impairments

Impairment in prerequisite communication skills includes impairment in social imitation. Autistic babies do not learn to wave "bye-bye;" they do not participate in imitative games like pat-a-cake, nor do they copy the routine actions of their parents (Fay & Schuler, 1980). They seem to have no organized system for thinking about past events, interpreting the present, and planning for the future. For the autistic child, things seem to happen in an apparently haphazard and random fashion (L. Wing, 1979). Defective organizational and symbolic skills preclude the acquisition of a system through which the child can learn from the environment. Autistic children demonstrate an absence of internal representation for external events that normally serves as a code to interpret the environment (Hermelin, 1978). Consequently, they are unable to learn to communicate by observing models in their environment. In order to recognize an object in a new context, the child must be able to process some new information from the context and compare it with some existing knowledge from previous experiences (Bloom & Lahey, 1978).

Autistic children are less likely to acquire communication skills through incidental learning (Litrownik, McInnis, Wetzel-Pritchard, & Filipelli, 1978) because they do not scan their environment and select relevant cues for learning (Koegel, Egel, & Dunlap, 1980). Rather, they select only a part of a relevant cue or respond to an insignificant aspect of the environment (Lovaas, Koegel, & Schreibman, 1979). It has been suggested that attention deficits account for the slowed or uneven learning rate of autistic children (Rincover, 1978). There is good evidence to suggest that autistic children focus their attention on only one aspect of a complex stimulus (Reynolds, Newsom, & Lovaas, 1974). The term applied to this phenomenon is *stimulus overselectivity*. It suggests that autistic children form discriminations on the basis of only one aspect or a peculiar combination of aspects of a stimulus (Lovaas, Schreibman, Koegel, & Rehm, 1971; Schreibman & Lovaas, 1973). Reynolds et al. (1974) suggest that auditory overselectivity may partially account for autistic deficits in speech comprehension.

The formulation of concepts is related to understanding the function of language (Cromer, 1981); thus, the cognitive processes that underlie the construction of a communication system is disturbed in autistic children (Dalgeish, 1975).

Sensory modulation and disturbances of perception in autistic children have been given considerable attention (Hermelin, 1978; Palkovitz & Wiesenfeld, 1980; Whetherby, Koegel, & Mendal, 1981). Eisenberg (1956) observed that "severely autistic children exhibit a preoccupation with sensory impressions stemming from the world about them, but seem unable to organize perceptions into functional patterns" (p. 611). Disturbances in relating may be a defense against incoming stimuli (Creak, 1972) or a result of faulty sensory modulation (Ornitz, 1974, 1978). Sensory impressions, particularly auditory sensations, are often distorted in autistic children. Some autistic children require a greater intensity of auditory input in order to perceive the stimulus (Mober & Simmons, 1981), whereas others seem to experience heightened sensitivity to sound (Menyuk, 1978). In contrast to aphasic children, who can respond appropriately to environmental noises other than speech long before they can understand and respond to speech (Eisenson, 1972), autistic children appear to ignore auditory stimuli in general but are alert to specific signals (Lowell, 1976), even though, as infants, they may show an unusual sensitivity to sound.

Other types of sensory and perceptual disturbances have been investigated in EEG studies that indicate a predominance of visual-spatial processing and a lack of dominance of auditory skills (Dawson, Warrenburg, & Fuller, 1982; O'Conner, 1971) and in studies on the reverberatory effects of auditory stimulation that may be associated with disordered perception and therefore with disturbances of speech, social relating, and movement (Condon, 1975; McGowan & Webster, 1980) and on the apparent inability to process rapidly occurring acoustic information (Tallal, 1976).

SUMMARY

Nearly 50 percent of autistic individuals are nonverbal; that is, they do not speak. The language behavior of those who do develop language, or speech, is strikingly different from that of individuals with other types of language disorders. Autistic children present a generalized lack of responsiveness in communicative contexts. They show gross deficits in language development, including disorders of syntax, semantics, and (in some cases) articulation. Even when their grammatical usage is correct, autistics do not seem to understand or use contextual cues for communication. Autistic speech is characterized by echolalic and stereotypic expressions, lacking spontaneity and abstraction. Pitch, stress, and intonation are unusual in the sense that rhythm is often either monotonic or sing-song. Pitch is either too high or too low, and, intensity is either too loud or too soft. Autistic individuals usually do not use gestures or facial expressions to facilitate meaning.

Paralinguistic social-communicative tools (bodily contact, proximity, orientation, appearance, posture, head nods, facial expressions, gestures, and looking) are lacking in the speech of the autistic person. Autistics seem to lack the ability to use symbols to interpret the environment and to convey messages to others. Other cognitive deficits—such as poor conceptual processing, stimulus overselectivity, inadequate sensory modulation, and disturbances of perception—may account for some of the disturbances in relating that are characteristic of autistic individuals.

Chapter 3

Managing Autistic Behavior

The emphasis of this manual is necessarily on the communicative aspects of autistic children's behavior. However, since communication does not occur in isolation, there are numerous other considerations in developing an approach to working with autistic children. Instructional procedures that approach the child as a whole being must account for multiple factors that have an impact on and, in turn, affect communicative behavior. One such consideration involves the necessity to examine behavioral characteristics that need to be changed and to design methods for dealing with problem behaviors.

The communication training of autistic children should be made an integral part of their world. A curriculum for teaching the most fundamental living skills can still emphasize communication; indeed, communication will underlie and pervade every aspect of instruction if the curriculum is well-planned. This requires careful and systematic control by the teacher or instructor. Any treatment program for autistic children must possess structure (Tanguay, 1976). This does not mean that the teacher must be an ogre, never crack a smile, or possess the qualities of a drill sergeant. On the contrary, it means that congeniality and fun have their place in the organized plan for helping autistic children reach their full potential. It has been demonstrated over and over again—and there is substantial evidence to support the conclusion—that a highly structured, data-based empirical approach is necessary (P. Clark & Rutter, 1981; Donnellan, 1980; Foxx, 1980a; Koegel & Egel, 1979; Ney, 1973). Schopler (1980) lists the following areas to be considered when designing structured educational settings:

- classroom organization and structure
- behavior management
- parent collaboration
- language training

- social skills development
- individualized developmental assessment
- individualized instruction
- individualized curricula
- prevocational/self-help skills

It should be noted that Schopler has included behavior management as a fundamental skill requirement for teachers of autistic children. This skill is necessary, not only for managing and controlling behaviors in the classroom and for preventing chaos, but also for analyzing tasks, organizing teaching processes, and determining child progress. In the following sections, we examine some of the techniques for managing behavior and for organizing instructional procedures.

THE TARGET BEHAVIOR

Webster's New Collegiate Dictionary (1981) defines behavior as a manner of conducting oneself. The term includes a complex set of observable and potentially measurable activities, including motor, cognitive, and physiological classes of responses to the environment (Bandura, 1969). The behavior manager is interested in developing habits, or in getting rid of unwanted habits. The empirical study of behavior involves examining the way an individual acts under given circumstances.

Behaviors can be expressed in terms of deficits or excesses (Gelfand & Hartmann, 1975). Behavioral "deficits" refer to those behaviors that are expected to be present for performing in a certain acceptable way but are, instead, absent. For example, one would expect a five-year-old child to be able to use a fork to eat meat. Some five-year-old autistic children do not use utensils for feeding. This is a behavior deficit, since the use of utensils is an expected behavior in five-year-olds. Behavioral excesses are behaviors that are inappropriate or interfere with the acquisition of important functional skills and that are present to a disturbing degree. A behavioral excess would be noted in the child who has tantrums every time the teacher requires the child to sit in a chair. Often, behavior management will require that excess behaviors, such as tantrums, be eliminated and that, simultaneously, new behaviors, such as sitting in a chair, be built in. Generally, a plan for teaching autistic children to be members of a community (even if the community consists solely of the classroom) must include an organized focus in both of these areas. The plan must be a systematic, structured one and must involve the careful programming of daily events in the child's life (Donnellan, 1980).

The first step in building new behaviors and eliminating inappropriate behaviors is to select the *target behavior*. The target behavior is the behavior (habit) that is selected for change. It can be either a behavioral deficit or a behavioral excess.

The target behavior will require a great deal of attention and concentration by the instructor. It is important to know exactly what the behavior is. Therefore, it must be defined in clear objective terms, so that it can be measured. For example, Mark spends most of his waking hours in self-stimulatory activity. Careful observation reveals that the self-stimulatory behavior consists primarily of twiddling his fingers in front of his face or lying on his back and pounding his heels on the floor. Mark's teacher wishes to change this behavior, so the target behavior is stated as "self-stimulation" and is defined (for Mark) as (1) twiddling his fingers in front of his face, and (2) lying on his back and pounding his heels on the floor. These behaviors are described well enough to be easily recognized. In addition, they can be measured, either by counting the number of times each self-stimulatory act occurs, or by totaling the amount of time spent in the self-stimulatory activity.

THE BASELINE

Before beginning a program to change the target behavior, it is important to observe the behavior and to record its frequency (Patterson, 1971). The best way for teachers or therapists to tell if their procedures are really working (changing the target behavior) is to measure it. The information obtained from a behavior-change program must be measured against a beginning point. This beginning point is known as the *baseline*. The systematic observation and recording of the target behavior prior to the beginning of intervention establishes a baseline. The baseline is the initial measurement of the behavior; it is an observation of how often and under what circumstances the behavior occurs. To return to the example of Mark's self-stimulatory behavior, the teacher takes a baseline measurement of Mark's "twiddling" and "pounding" by recording on a chart each time the behavior occurs. If the teacher wishes to ascertain more information about the circumstances surrounding the behavior, this can be marked on the chart.

An example of a baseline chart for Mark's self-stimulatory behavior is shown in Exhibit 3–1. Notice that the teacher has divided the chart into sections denoting each hour of the school day. In this way, the teacher can determine whether or not the self-stimulation occurs more frequently at certain times during the day. The teacher has also noted on the chart

Exhibit 3–1 Baseline Chart for Mark's Self-Stimulatory Behavior

Target Behavior: Mark's self-stimulatory behavior (twiddling fingers in front of his eyes; lying on his back and pounding his heels on the floor)

Baseline: 116 (Total for 5 days)

Time:	9:00	10:00	11:00	12:00	1:00	2:00	3:00	Total
Activity:	Language Group	Individual Attend	Individual Self-help	Lunch	Gym	Individual Language	Group Music	
Monday	111	1	11	~~1111~~	~~1111~~ 11	11	111	23
Tuesday	1111	11	11	~~1111~~ 111	1111	1	~~1111~~ ~~1111~~	31
Wednesday	1111	1	111	~~1111~~	111	111	~~1111~~ 1	25
Thursday	1		11	1111	~~1111~~	1	1111	17
Friday	1	11		~~1111~~	1111	111	~~1111~~	20
							Total for week:	116

the various activities that occur during each hour so that it can be determined if some activities may be related to the self-stimulatory behavior in some way. Such information could be important in choosing a program for decreasing the self-stimulatory behavior.

The baseline chart for Mark's self-stimulatory behavior shows that it is indeed a high-rate behavior (occurs frequently) and that it seems to occur more often in group activities and less often in individual settings. The teacher does not, at this point, make any assumptions about why the behavior occurs more or less frequently at such times. However, when a behavior change program is initiated the effectiveness of the intervention procedures will be measured against the baseline measurements in these same settings.

Obtaining an accurate baseline requires that the behavior be recorded *every* time it occurs. It is also very important to refrain from intervening in the behavior when establishing the baseline. Though it is tempting to try to stop the behavior before a planned procedure has been developed, particularly if the behavior is one that annoys the teacher, the accuracy or reliability of the baseline depends upon how well the teacher can *ignore* the behavior while counting it. (This does not hold true, of course, if the behavior is one that is harmful to the child or to others.) (An extra baseline chart form is provided in Appendix A for teacher use.)

INCREASING THE TARGET BEHAVIOR

Reinforcement

Whether we like it or not, there are consequences of almost everything we do. People who show up an hour late for work every morning are likely to lose their jobs. Losing one's job is a consequence of showing up late. Children who eat ice cream, cake, candy, and soda pop at a party are likely to have a stomachache afterwards. A stomachache is the consequence of eating ice cream, cake, candy, and soda pop. On the other hand, a worker who arrives on time for all meetings and consistently pleases the boss may receive a pay raise. The pay raise is the consequence of appropriate behavior (arriving at meetings on time and pleasing the boss) at work. Most of us try to avoid unpleasant consequences, such as stomachaches; we are encouraged by the consequences to keep our inappropriate behavior at a minimum. We also try to accumulate pleasant consequences, such as earning a pay raise, by increasing our production of behaviors that seem to get us those pleasant consequences. The same principle applies to the process of teaching autistic children. Teachers use consequences to encourage appropriate behaviors and to discourage inappropriate behaviors.

Consequences are events that follow a behavior and either increase or decrease the behavior. Reinforcement is a type of consequence that follows a behavior and maintains or increases it. For example, every time Peggy says "cookie," the teacher gives her a bit of cookie. Over a period of one week, Peggy increases the number of times she says "cookie" from 2 times on Monday to 55 times on Friday. Thus, it can be demonstrated that the bit of cookie that Peggy received every time she said "cookie" was a reinforcer for saying "cookie." It should be remembered that reinforcers (1) follow a behavior and (2) strengthen the behavior that they follow.

Reinforcement can be enhanced by combining it with the target behavior in the instructional setting. An experiment by Koegel and Williams (1980) illustrates this principle. They compared the performance of autistic children in two different learning conditions. In the first, the target behavior was a direct part of the chain leading to the reinforcer, for example, opening the lid of a container to obtain a food reward inside the container. In the second, the target behavior was an indirect part of the chain leading to the reinforcer, for example, the therapist handing the child a food reward after the child had opened the lid of an empty container. Koegel and Williams found that a more rapid acquisition of the target behavior occurred when it was a direct part of the chain.

Reinforcers come in all sizes and shapes, but they are generally classified as either social reinforcers or backup reinforcers. Social reinforcement involves the teacher's behavior toward the child, for example, tone of voice, words of praise, giving attention, touching, hugging, and being near the child (Becker, Engelmann, & Thomas, 1971). Backup reinforcement backs up or fortifies social reinforcement. Backup reinforcers can be food reinforcers, token reinforcers (points, poker chips, money, and so on, that can be exchanged for a more valuable commodity), or activity reinforcers (games, walks in the park, and so forth). Activity reinforcers are often referred to as "grandma's rule" (or the Premack Principle), which says, "First, you do what I want you to do, then you can do what you want to do" (Becker, 1971; Becker et al., 1971). Teachers and therapists may find it helpful to use a chart like that in Exhibit 3–2 to list reinforcers that will later be useful in increasing newly trained behaviors in autistic children.

Schedules of Reinforcement

Reinforcement may be given following every occurrence of the target behavior, or it may be given periodically. If reinforcement is given after

Exhibit 3–2 Chart for Listing Reinforcers in Teaching Autistic Children

Reinforcement List		
Social Reinforcers:	**Backup Reinforcers:**	
_____	**Edible Reinforcers:**	
_____	_____ _____	
_____	_____ _____	
_____	_____ _____	
_____	_____ _____	
_____	_____ _____	
_____	**Activity Reinforcers:**	
_____	_____ _____	
_____	_____ _____	
_____	_____ _____	
_____	_____ _____	
	_____ _____	
	Token Reinforcers:	
	_____ _____	
	_____ _____	
	_____ _____	
	_____ _____	
	_____ _____	

each occurrence of the behavior, it is called *continuous*. If it is given periodically, it is called *intermittent* (Smith & Moore, 1966). A continuous reinforcement schedule usually results in more rapid acquisition of the behavior. Thus, if the teacher or therapist wishes to quickly establish or increase the target behavior, reinforcement will be given each time the behavior is observed. Sometimes, however, it is desirable to use an intermittent schedule of reinforcement, for example, in cases where, once the new behavior has been well-established, the teacher wishes to maintain the behavior over a long period of time.

Intermittent schedules of reinforcement can be of two types: ratio or interval. A ratio schedule means that the behavior is reinforced as a function of the number of responses or occurrences. The teacher may decide to reinforce the child either on a fixed-ratio (FR) schedule (a fixed number of responses is reinforced) or on a variable (VR) schedule (the number of responses that are reinforced is variable). An interval schedule means that the behavior is reinforced as a function of time. For example, the teacher may decide to reinforce the behavior every 15 minutes or every minute, as long as the target behavior is occurring. Interval schedules can also be fixed (FI) or variable (VI).

How To Use Reinforcement

The following procedures will help make reinforcement more effective:

- *Select the reinforcement carefully.* Try to choose reinforcers that have been demonstrated to "work" with a particular child. Observe the child to see which food items, games, or toys are most frequently chosen. Ask parents and other significant adults to make a list of the child's known likes and dislikes. Experiment (try out different things) to see what seems to motivate the child.
- *Avoid giving the child too much of a good thing.* Combine several reinforcers, such as social ("That's right!") and backup edible (a sip of juice). Vary the reinforcer. The use of the same reinforcer over and over again can reduce effectiveness.
- *Make the reinforcement contingent upon the desired performance.* Make sure the child gives the correct response or the desired behavior *before* the reinforcer is given. Giving the reinforcement and then trying to coax the child to produce the desired behavior may teach the child to postpone producing the desired response. It may also reinforce the child for *not* producing the desired behavior.
- *Reinforce immediately.* As soon as the child emits the desired behavior, reinforce it. This tells the child exactly which behavior was the right one, and it decreases the possibility that an inappropriate behavior will "slip in" and accidentally be reinforced.
- *Reinforce every correct response or occurrence when new behaviors are being established.* Gradually shift to intermittent schedules as target behaviors become habits.
- *Make sure the reinforcement is under the teacher's control.* The child should have access to the reinforcer only when the desired behavior has occurred.
- *Make sure that the reinforcement is practical.* Walking around the school building may be a strong reinforcer for a particular child, but it is impractical in a setting where the target behavior may occur several times an hour.
- *The reinforcement should be compatible with the program.* A five-pound box of chocolates would not be a compatible reinforcement for the child who is on a weight-loss program.

Prompting

Prompts are the primary tools to establish new behaviors (Foxx, 1980a). They are used to shape, or gradually teach, behaviors that were previously absent. They have been demonstrated to be very effective in teaching communication skills to disabled children (Weaver & Ruder, 1978). The key idea is that prompting involves physically guiding the child through the steps in completing a new task. If, for example, Lucy is unable to use utensils to feed herself, the instructor could provide a prompt to teach her the new behavior. The instructor would prompt Lucy by placing a spoon in her hand, then, physically guiding her hand to scoop food from the plate and into her mouth.

Motivating autistic children has long been considered an essential part of the instructional process (Koegel et al., 1980; Rutter, 1978b). Considerable attention has been given to investigating motivational factors. It has been suggested that failure to succeed affects the motivation of autistic children. Prompting is an effective tool in motivating autistic children to complete a task (Koegel & Egel, 1979). When children are prompted successfully to complete a task, such as buttoning, the rate of reinforcement increases. Koegel and Egel (1979) have demonstrated that increases in reinforcement produce the desirable effects of strengthening motivation, particularly for autistic children whose behavioral repertoire is severely depleted.

Prompts are very much like a crutch. They are essential for the person who has a broken leg, for, without them, that person could not walk. It could be said that the crutch does the walking for the person. People can become dependent upon crutches, however, and they should be discarded as soon as the person becomes able to walk alone. Similarly, autistic children can become dependent upon prompts. Therefore, it is important to fade prompts as soon as possible so that the child will learn to perform the behavior independently. Prompt fading is the gradual withdrawal of prompts. It is accomplished by providing lots of guidance for the child at first, then systematically and gradually decreasing the amount of help given. Prompts may be faded by reducing the physical guidance from a full touch to a partial touch, or by reducing the full touch to a gesture or some other visual cue.

Modeling

Modeling may be considered a kind of prompt because it involves giving the child a clue about the expected behavior. It is considered separately here, however, for purposes of clarity. Modeling teaches a new behavior by allowing the child to observe the teacher or therapist perform the desired behavior (J.D. Krumboltz & H.B. Krumboltz, 1972). In this instructional procedure, the instructor demonstrates the desired behavior, such as showing the manual sign for milk. When the child produces the sign for milk, the instructor reinforces it.

Prompting and modeling can be combined when it is desirable to teach a new behavior more rapidly or when a child is unable to replicate the behavior by observing it. To combine prompting and modeling, the instructor begins by modeling the desired behavior, for example, by showing the manual sign for food. The instructor then takes the child's hand and shapes it into the sign (prompting). The prompts are then gradually faded by giving decreasing amounts of physical guidance for the sign, so that the child eventually forms the sign for food in response to the model. (An example of combining prompting, modeling, and prompt fading is shown in an attending program in Chapter 5.)

Successive Approximations

Sometimes children are not able to complete a task correctly, but they are able to perform parts of the task, or are able to begin the task. The principle of successive approximation involves rewarding or reinforcing successive steps to the final behavior (J.D. Krumboltz & H.B. Krumboltz, 1972). This teaching technique requires that complex skills be broken down into small steps that can be reinforced as the child comes closer and closer to the desired behavior. For example, as a first step in learning to produce the sound /m/, Dwight is reinforced for putting his lips together. This is an approximation of the desired behavior. Later, Dwight puts his lips together and grunts. This is a closer approximation to the sound /m/, so Dwight is reinforced for this. Finally, Dwight puts his lips together and emits a distinct /m/. At this point, he is reinforced for the /m/ sound, but he is not reinforced for repetitions of the previous approximations.

Teaching a new skill by successive approximations begins by requiring the child to produce a response that is within the range of the child's ability and is at least remotely related to the goal or target behavior. The program then moves in gradual steps so that correct responses are more likely to occur and each response brings the child closer to the goal (Costello, 1977).

DECREASING THE TARGET BEHAVIOR

Extinction

There are several ways of decreasing the target behavior. The first involves the use of extinction. Extinction means that the instructor no longer provides a reinforcer following a particular behavior (Bandura, 1969). When extinction is used, the behavior that was previously reinforced generally decreases, sometimes after a temporary increase in the behavior (extinction burst) (Gelfand & Hartmann, 1975). In order for extinction to be effective, the teacher must know what the reinforcer is and must be able to control it by withholding it. It is easy to assume that all one need do is to withhold attention and the child will cease the inappropriate behavior. Attention from the adult may well be the reinforcer that is maintaining much child behavior; however, the teacher must examine other possibilities, especially with autistic children. For example, attention from peers may be maintaining the behavior; if so, it will be difficult for the teacher to control this reinforcer.

The use of extinction should follow these four guidelines:

1. The instructor should avoid looking at the child while the inappropriate behavior is occurring. Eye contact can be socially reinforcing for some children. Even though autistic children do not voluntarily give social eye contact, there is the possibility that this form of attention from an adult could be reinforcing.
2. The instructor should avoid calling attention to the behavior. This also could be a way of providing social reinforcement for the child.
3. The instructor should continue working with the child in a "business-as-usual" manner, carefully avoiding giving any type of reinforcement to the target behavior.
4. Extinction should be used with behaviors that have previously been reinforced. When used in this manner, the effect of the withheld reinforcer will be stronger.

Punishment

An event that follows a behavior and decreases or eliminates it is called punishment. The teacher or therapist must remember that the definitions given here for reinforcement and punishment are operant definitions; that is, the processes are defined operationally, in terms of their effect on a behavior. Placing value judgments on reinforcement (something "good") and punishment (something "bad") is an error in behavior management. If a behavior increases or stays at a steady rate, it is being reinforced. If a behavior decreases or stops, it is being punished. Suppose, for example, that, every time Tommy pinches the teacher, he is placed in a chair in the corner of the room for three minutes. Tommy stops pinching the teacher Being placed in a chair in the corner for three minutes actually punished the pinching behavior. Suppose, on the other hand, that, every time Tommy pinches the teacher, he is sent to the principal's office. Tommy continues to pinch the teacher. Being sent to the principal's office did not actually punish the pinching behavior.

Startle Response

A relatively mild form of punishment that is used to interrupt a disruptive behavior is the startle response. Robinson, Hughes, Wilson, Lahey, and Haynes (1974) used water squirts to effectively reduce self-stimulatory behavior in autistic children. The water squirt was also used to reduce aggressive behavior in a retarded boy (Gross, Berler, & Drabman, 1982). Generally, however, the startle response involves a sudden loud noise such as "no!" or a bright flash of light. The startle is not intended to harm the child, nor to cause discomfort. Rather, it is intended to surprise the child so that the inappropriate or disruptive behavior ceases immediately.

The following guidelines will make the use of the startle response more effective:

- Interrupt the behavior with a sudden response. Do not wait until the behavior has stopped.
- Avoid making eye contact with the child prior to and immediately following the startle. If eye contact is made prior to the startle, the child may get a clue about what will happen next and the startle effect will be diminished. If eye contact is made immediately following the startle, the child may derive some social reinforcement from the "game."
- After a few seconds following the startle, give the child an alternative appropriate behavior to do, so that reinforcement can be given for the alternative behavior.

Overcorrection

Since Chapter 4 examines the subject of overcorrection in some detail, it will be dealt with only briefly here. Recently, overcorrection has been used extensively to control and redirect behaviors of autistic and other severely developmentally delayed children (Axelrod, Brantner, & Meddock, 1978; Azrin, Gottlieb, Hugart, Wesolowski, & Rahn, 1975; Czyzewski, Barrera, & Sulzer-Azaroff, 1982). Overcorrection involves repeated practice designed to decrease a problem behavior.

Timeout

Timeout means the withdrawal of the situation in which reinforcement occurs (Reese, 1966). This is generally accomplished by removing the child from a reinforcing environment or by removing the opportunity for positive reinforcement. It also includes the removal of the opportunity to receive positive reinforcement for a specified period of time (Sulzer-Aza-roff & Mayer, 1977). It has been demonstrated that timeout can be an effective method for controlling disruptive and inappropriate behaviors in autistic children (Wolf, Risley, & Mees, 1964). However, the teacher or therapist working with autistic children must base decisions to use timeout on the individual characteristics of each autistic child. For some autistic children, isolation may be reinforcing (Becker et al., 1971); for others, it may be too frightening.

Various Forms

There are different ways of removing the opportunity to receive rein-forcement. As stated above, timeout can be the removal of the child from the environment or it can be the removal of access to reinforcing activities. Either way, the principle of timeout requires that no reinforcement be available for a specified period of time. Removal of the child to an area or room where there is nothing to do is one way to accomplish timeout. The child may also be required to sit in a chair and not participate in an activity. Another way to use timeout is for the teacher or therapist to restrain the child physically by holding the child in a chair.

Removal of the child from the environment has the advantage of ensuring that other children and adults will not accidentally reinforce the child by their nearness or by talking to the child. For most children, removal has the added advantage of ensuring that the child has nothing reinforcing to do. With autistic children, however, there is no such insurance policy. In many cases, the autistic child seems to take advantage of the situation by seizing the opportunity to engage in self-stimulatory behavior while no one will interrupt. Certainly, timeout will not be effective with such children. An additional precaution must be taken with children who are removed to a timeout booth or room. In this case, the teacher or therapist must be able to observe the child at all times so that, in cases of self-injury or accidental injury, the child can be removed from the timeout situation at once. In such cases, an alternative punishment will have to be found.

Requiring a child to sit on a chair in a corner of the room or away from the reinforcing activity has the advantage of being a somewhat milder form of punishment than removal to a timeout booth or room. Also, in the cases of children who are somewhat social, this form of timeout has the added advantage of "showing" the children what they are missing. The point is that, as with all forms of timeout, the environment or activity from which the child is removed must be highly reinforcing; otherwise, the timeout will not be punishing. Removal to a chair is also preferable in classrooms where there is one teacher and several students, because it does not require that the teacher leave the classroom to accompany the child to timeout and then remain in the timeout area to observe the child.

The disadvantages of removing a child to a chair are obvious. First, the opportunity to observe the activities or even to hear the goings-on may be as reinforcing as participation. The teacher must know, in advance, the peculiarities of the child. Second, it may be difficult to control other children and to keep them from interacting with the child being "timed out." Third, the teacher must expect that some children will not remain in the timeout area or chair unless they are restrained. Again, the effectiveness of this type of timeout will depend upon the particular child and upon the teacher's or therapist's control of the situation.

Restraint alleviates the possibility of the child getting out of the chair; however, it also requires the full-time presence of the adult, and this may be impractical in a classroom situation. Restraint also poses a problem because it involves physical contact with the child. Some children enjoy the physical contact, so this can be potentially reinforcing. Even a child who struggles against the physical contact or restraint may be reinforced in such a situation during the timeout period. One way of overcoming inadvertent reinforcement during such times is to use a procedure called quiet training (Foxx, 1980a). In this procedure, the teacher or therapist physically directs the child to lie on the floor, face up, and physically restrains the limbs. The teacher avoids looking at or talking to the child. The teacher releases the physical restraint as the child calms down; and, after about one minute of quiet behavior, the child is allowed to return to the activity. The size and strength of the student (and the teacher) will partially determine whether or not this type of timeout procedure should be used.

Guidelines

The following procedures and guidelines will help make the use of timeout more effective:

- As soon as the target behavior occurs, lead the child by the wrist, or direct the child from behind, to the designated timeout area (chair, booth, room). Guidance from behind or assistance from another adult may be necessary for a very resistive or aggressive autistic child.
- Do not engage in power struggles with the child. Ask for assistance from another adult or physically restrain the child until the aggression ceases, then proceed to the timeout area.

- Name the behavior for which the child is being timed out. For example, "That's hitting. Time out." Even autistic children who do not seem to understand verbal directions should be given the benefit of being told what they are being punished for.
- Proceed to the timeout area in a calm, unemotional manner. Avoid giving the child a chance to be reinforced by upsetting the adult and avoid displaying anger. Avoid emotional outbursts that may result in accidental harm to the child.
- Do not scold, argue, or yell. Once the offensive behavior has been stated, refrain from further verbal interaction with the child.
- Avoid making eye contact with the child on the way to the timeout area. Again, eye contact can be a potential source of reinforcement.
- Calmly place the child in the timeout area.
- Record the date, the behavior for which the child is being timed out, the time the child was placed in the timeout area, the behavior during timeout, and the time the child was taken out or released from timeout (see the sample timeout log in Exhibit 3–3).
- At all times remain close enough to the timeout area to observe the child. If the child becomes self-abusive, remove the child from the area at once.
- After the designated period of timeout (usually about one minute, but never longer than five to ten minutes), lead the child back to the activity or direct the child to complete the interrupted task. Avoid scolding, or making such remarks as, "I hope you're ready to behave now."
- Make sure that the environment is rewarding by providing a high degree of reinforcement. If the environment is not reinforcing, the child may seek to escape by being sent to timeout.
- Use timeout every time the target behavior occurs, and as soon as it occurs. If the child starts the behavior, then anticipates timeout and stops the behavior, timeout should be implemented anyway.
- Ignore all protests or promises of, "I won't do it again."
- Use timeout only for the behavior that has been targeted and specified for timeout. Do not shift to another procedure until the behavior is under control or until it has been established that timeout is ineffective for a particular child.

Other Forms of Punishment

The most serious kinds of behavior, such as self-injury, can be effectively treated with aversive means. Electric stimulation ("shock") has been used to treat such deviant forms of behavior as self-mutilation (Lovaas,

Exhibit 3–3 Sample Timeout Log

Timeout Log				
Date	Target Behavior	Time "In"	Behavior during Timeout	Time "Out"

Schaeffer, & Simmons, 1965; Risley, 1968). This type of punishment is rarely used; it is in fact forbidden in many settings because of the potential for abuse and possible harmful side effects. In any case, it should never be used by anyone other than a trained professional with thorough review and monitoring by a panel of experts.

Another form of aversive treatment, physical punishment, such as a slap on the leg, has been used effectively with autistic children (Bucher & Lovaas, 1968; Koegel & Covert, 1972; Lovaas, 1981). Because it is a model for aggression, however, physical punishment is generally reserved for extreme cases, such as self-injury or harmful self-stimulation. All of the considerations for the use of electric stimulation apply to the use of physical punishment. It should be used only by trained professionals, it should be used only in extreme cases, it should be carefully monitored, and parental and legal consent must be obtained. Also, it must be empirically demonstrated that other, less aversive, means have failed to reduce the behavior, and that allowing the target behavior to continue would actually have greater harmful effects than any possible side effects produced by the punishment procedure.

Ethical Considerations

Teachers and therapists who design and implement punishment procedures must be aware of the potential dangers involved in such procedures, as well as the advantages of using them, and must take the necessary precautionary steps to avoid the dangers. Punishing children is not something that adults readily enjoy, and public protest may be aroused when it appears that a child, particularly a handicapped one, is being "abused." The conscientious behavior manager knows that, when punishment is used appropriately, it is much less harmful to the child than it would be to allow the inappropriate behavior to continue. Nevertheless, conscientious teachers and therapists are continually under fire from well-meaning, but misguided, observers. A few precautionary guidelines will help alleviate some of the misunderstanding:

- The explicit procedures for the use of punishment, and the specific behavior for which the punishment will be used should be carefully thought out and written down.
- Parental or guardian consent should be obtained, in writing, before the punishment procedure is implemented.
- The punishment procedure should be conducted openly and its effects should be carefully evaluated by professionals, using accurate data recording and analysis procedures.
- Punishment should be used when positive reinforcement alone has proven ineffective; and the milder forms of punishment should be used first, before using more aversive procedures.
- The child should be given optimal opportunity to receive positive reinforcement in the educational environment.

Punishment can be a most effective treatment model for dealing with inappropriate behaviors. It produces immediate and complete suppression of the behavior when it is implemented correctly (Foxx, 1980b). However, punishment also has disadvantages associated with producing emotional stress and anxiety. That is why it is imperative that the teacher or therapist follow the above guidelines in designing and implementing any punishment procedure.

The most important rule in the use of any punishment procedure is to provide a proper balance of reinforcement for positive behaviors. Sometimes that is easier said than done, particularly with autistic children. Teachers and therapists thus must become astute observers of subtle behavior so that they can "catch" the child doing something appropriate. The child may at first need additional guidance or prompting. When the child cooperates or begins to perform a task without help, the teacher should seize the moment to heap rewards upon the child. The therapist can request the child to do something the child can (and will!) do, even if it means asking the child to take a bite of a favorite food. The child in this case has complied with the therapist's request, and can be reinforced. Unless a reinforcing environment is provided, chances are that the child will be overly punished, become "hardened" to the punishment, increase the inappropriate behavior, and require more aversive methods of controlling the behavior. Punishment then loses its effectiveness. An aversive environment is not a pretty sight; however, it can easily be avoided by providing the proper amount of reinforcement at the proper times.

MEASURING PROGRESS

Collecting Data

The purpose of collecting data is to provide a continuous record of child progress and to detect ineffective treatment procedures so that changes can be made (Gelfand & Hartmann, 1975). The importance of establishing a baseline was discussed earlier in this chapter. The baseline shows the frequency of the behavior before consequences are implemented. Once the consequences have been selected, a means for measuring the effect of the consequences on the target behavior must be established. Ways of measuring behavior were discussed as a part of measuring the baseline; however, some further suggestions can be made here.

As we have noted, data can be collected either by counting the number of occurrences of the behavior or by totaling the amount of time spent in the behavior. Data are also collected during instructional sessions. During these sessions, the responses of the child are recorded as correct or incorrect, and the percentage of correct responses is figured at the end of the session. (A more detailed explanation of these recording procedures is included in Chapter 5 in the instructions for teaching the child to attend.)

The chart in Exhibit 3–4 shows how the data for a target behavior may be collected. (An extra chart form for teacher use is provided in Appendix A.) In this example, the number of occurrences is tabulated so that the effects of the intervention (consequence) can be analyzed. The data are

Exhibit 3–4 Chart for Recording Behavioral Change Data

BEHAVIOR CHANGE CHART

Target Behavior: *Mark's self-stimulatory behavior*

Baseline: *116 (Total for 5 days)*

Consequence: *overcorrection*

Time	9:00	10:00	11:00	12:00	1:00	2:00	3:00		
Activity	Language Group	Indiv. Attend.	Indiv. Selfhelp	Lunch	Gym	Indiv. Lang.	Group Music		
Date									Total
9-18	///	/	//	THL	THL I	///	////		24
9-19	//	//	/	///	//	/	///		14
9-20	/	///	//	/	///	//	/		13
9-21	//	/	/	THL	THL II	/	THL		22
9-22	/	//	/	II	/	/	///		11
9-25	//	///	////	THL	///	/	THL		23
9-26	/	/	//	/	/	/	///		10
9-27			/	///	//		//		8
9-28				THL	II		/		8
9-29				/			/		2

of no use unless they are analyzed. Analysis involves examining the data and comparing them with the baseline. The data must show that the behavior is changing in the desired direction, either increasing or decreasing. If the behavior is not changing, or if it is changing in the wrong direction, this is a signal that the program is not working and changes must be made in the program itself.

Graphing Data

It is always helpful if the instructor can glance at the data and determine if the child is making progress. A behavioral graph is a tool to aid the instructor in analyzing the data; it is a pictorial representation of the child's progress. Each plot on the graph represents one unit of data. The graph in Figure 3–1 shows how data can be plotted to show the direction of behavior change. The graph presents the baseline data from Exhibit 3–1 and the sample data from Exhibit 3–4. Notice how effectively the graph demonstrates the behavior change that has taken place as a result of the

Figure 3–1 Graph of Behavior Change

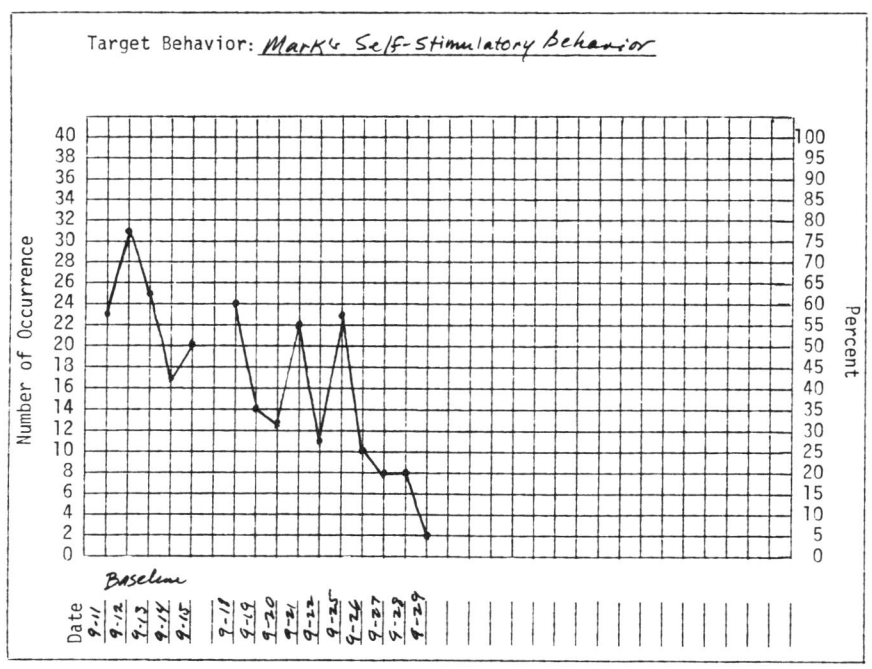

intervention (consequence). (An extra graph form for teacher use is provided in Appendix A.)

PROGRAMMING NEW BEHAVIORS

So far, we have concentrated on ways of increasing and decreasing behaviors, and we have described ways to aid children in developing new behaviors (prompting, modeling, successive approximation). The effectiveness of these procedures will depend upon how well the teacher or instructor understands the learning process underlying the development of an instructional program. The development of instructional programs for teaching autistic children new tasks requires some special skills. One of these skills is task analysis.

New skills are learned more easily if they are broken down into very tiny, simple steps (L. Wing, 1972). Task analysis is "breaking down a complex skill or behavioral chain into its component behaviors, sub-skills, or sub-tasks. Each component is stated in its order of occurrence and sets the occasion for the occurrence of the next behavior" (Sulzer-Azaroff & Mayer, 1977, p. 524).

Task analysis is most often used to break down the complex skills involved in teaching severely handicapped and retarded children to perform, with minimum error, the complex skills involved in self-help (feeding, dressing, and so forth), communication, perceptual motor activities (gross and fine motor activities, physical education, and so on), and socialization. (For complete programs in these areas, see Baldwin, Fredericks, & Brodsky, 1973, and Popovitch & Laham, 1981.)

Uneven task performance is typical in autistic children (M.K. DeMyer et al., 1971). For example, a child may be able to reach for the soap and lather up the hands for washing but not be able to turn the faucet on. Such uneven skill development again points to the necessity to break down complex skills (such as hand-washing) into small, sequential steps.

The focus of any instructional program for autistic children should take into account the interaction of behaviors that sometimes appear to be unrelated. While we are not sure to what extent autistic children's communication deficits affect behavior, and vice versa, we do know that the establishment of behavioral control is the first step in teaching these children anything, and that the second step is a planned, systematic instructional program.

SUMMARY

It has been demonstrated that a highly structured, data-based program is most suitable for autistic children. Behavior management is a fundamental skill requirement for teachers of autistic children. Not only must teachers be able to control problem behaviors, they must also be able to analyze and measure progress on tasks that are taught.

Behavior may be classed as behavioral deficits or behavioral excesses. Behavioral deficits are those behaviors that are absent but the child should have. Behavioral excesses are inappropriate behaviors that occur with undesirable frequency. The optimal educational setting will systematically reduce excess behaviors and build in behaviors that are deficit.

Teachers use consequences to strengthen appropriate behaviors and to weaken or eliminate inappropriate ones. Reinforcement is a general term for the class of consequences that follow a behavior and strengthen or increase the behavior. Punishment is the term used to describe consequences that decrease or eliminate the behavior. Shaping new behaviors involves the use of reinforcement and punishment, as well as prompting (giving lots of help), prompt fading, modeling (demonstrating), and reinforcement of successive approximations (gradually increasing the criterion as the child comes closer and closer to the expected response). Decreasing undesirable behaviors involves the careful and ethical use of punishment procedures, such as extinction, startle response, overcorrection, timeout, and, in extremely rare cases, physical punishment. The most important rule in the use of punishment procedures is to provide a proper balance of reinforcement for positive behaviors.

The target behavior is the behavior that will be changed in some way (eliminated or taught). The systematic observation and recording of the target behavior prior to intervention is called establishing the baseline. The effectiveness of the intervention is measured by collecting and analyzing the data.

Chapter 4

Overcorrection

Several procedures for decreasing inappropriate behaviors were discussed in Chapter 3. Extinction and punishment procedures—such as the startle response, timeout, aversives, and physical punishment—have been effective in reducing and eliminating problem behaviors, but they also are complicated by potential harmful or unpleasant side effects. Unless programs for reducing behaviors are carefully planned, punishment procedures can have negative effects. Such procedures do not, of themselves, teach children appropriate behaviors as alternatives to the inappropriate ones, nor do they teach children new skills. It is possible to envision an autistic child whose treatment has effectively eliminated all self-stimulatory behavior but who has nothing appropriate to do instead. All too often, the result is a child who is a motoric "zombie," or the child develops other self-stimulatory behaviors or inappropriate behaviors to take the place of the behaviors that were extinguished. To avoid such unfortunate consequences of punishment, meticulous planning for functional skill development and scrupulous attention to reinforcement for appropriate behaviors are critical. Punishment procedures do not generally have built-in mechanisms for such constructive teaching. The teacher must be alert and adept at following through with reinforcement of appropriate behaviors that are incompatible with the inappropriate behavior being punished.

There is, however, a recently developed technique that combines reductive procedures (punishment) with reeducative procedures (instruction). This procedure, developed by Foxx and Azrin (1972), is called overcorrection.

The principle of overcorrection states that inappropriate behaviors can be treated by required practice in the appropriate behavior whenever the former behavior appears (Azrin, Kaplan, & Foxx, 1973). Overcorrection seems to involve some characteristics of reductive, as well as productive, techniques, such as timeout, punishment, and skill building (Gaylord-

59

Ross, 1980). The underlying mechanism that gives overcorrection its potency as a punishment procedure is not yet known. However, in many cases it is more effective than physical punishment, extinction, or reinforcement for not engaging in inappropriate behaviors (Foxx & Azrin, 1973a).

EXAMPLES OF THE USE OF OVERCORRECTION

Overcorrection has been shown to be effective in eliminating various forms of self-stimulatory behavior in retarded and autistic individuals. Foxx and Azrin (1973a) demonstrated the effectiveness of overcorrection procedures in reducing self-stimulatory behaviors of three retarded children and one autistic child. The self-stimulatory behaviors exhibited by the children were object-mouthing, hand-mouthing, head-weaving and hand-clapping. The overcorrection method for mouthing objects and for hand-mouthing was the "oral hygiene procedure" (Foxx & Azrin, 1972), which had previously been used to reduce aggressive biting in a retarded adult and a brain-damaged adult. The procedure consisted of telling the child, "No," in a firm voice, then directing the child to brush her gums and teeth with a toothbrush that had been soaked in an oral antiseptic (mouthwash). The child was directed to wipe her lips with a washcloth that had been dampened with the mouthwash. Each administration of the oral hygiene procedure was conducted for a period of two minutes.

The overcorrection procedure for head-weaving was "functional movement training." This consisted of instructing and manually guiding the child to move her head in one of three positions—up, down, or straight— in random order. This overcorrection procedure was conducted for a period of five minutes.

The overcorrection procedure for hand-clapping also involved functional movement training. The child was required to engage in five minutes of moving his hands in various positions: above his head, straight out in front of him, into his pockets, held together, and held behind his back. He was required to hold his hands in each position for 15 seconds, following the instruction given by the teacher.

These overcorrection procedures were compared with (1) free reinforcement, in which the child was reinforced with candy and cereal at regular intervals; (2) reinforcement for nonmouthing, in which reinforcement was given for each ten-second interval of nonmouthing behavior; (3) an aversive punishment procedure, in which a slap on the thigh was given each time the child engaged in mouthing; and (4) a distasteful solution (a commercially available solution to discourage thumb-sucking in normal children) that was painted on the child's hand. It was found that the overcorrection procedures produced more rapid and longer-lasting reduction of the self-stimulatory behavior.

In an expanded study (Azrin et al., 1973), body-rocking, head-weaving, hand movements, and complex finger movements of 32 institutionalized retarded individuals were eliminated by a combination of overcorrection procedures similar to those described above (Foxx & Azrin, 1973a) and reinforcement for using recreational and educative materials appropriately. The overcorrection procedures consisted of telling the resident, "No! don't rock" (the instructor specifically stated the inappropriate behavior). Then the instructor stood behind the resident and directed positive practice movements topographically related to the self-stimulatory behavior. The resident was required to practice the overcorrection procedure for 20 minutes.

The oral hygiene procedure (brushing the teeth with an oral antiseptic) was also used to eliminate thumb-sucking during language instruction (Doke & Epstein, 1975). In this study, it was found that the reduction of thumb-sucking could be maintained by verbal threats or warnings. However, the suppression of thumb-sucking did not generalize to other settings when only verbal threats were used. Also, when thumb-sucking was eliminated by overcorrection during other activities, other nonoral misbehaviors appeared and increased.

In another study, the combined effects of reduced self-stimulatory behavior and the acquisition of an appropriate functional skill were demonstrated by Wells, Forehand, Hickey, and Green (1977). Stereotypic behaviors were reversed when the subject was required to practice appropriate toy play.

Rollings, A.A. Baumeister, and A.A. Baumeister (1977) effectively reduced body-rocking by making practice in the correct behavior contingent upon the self-stimulatory behavior. The positive effects of overcorrection in this study, however, did not generalize to other (nontreatment) settings, nor did the suppression of body-rocking endure over a period of six months.

Overcorrection procedures not topographically related to self-stimulatory behavior have also been found to be effective. Roberts, Iwata, McSween, and Desmond (1979) reduced the stereotypic behaviors (mouthing, grabbing, hand-clapping, head-wagging, growling, running material or skin between the fingers, screaming, masturbation, facial grimacing, and hitting objects) of three retarded adults by verbally instructing or manually guiding them to engage in repeated exercises for a specified period of time. The required exercises were not necessarily related to the self-stimulatory behavior. For example, mouthing objects was punished by requiring the subject to practice repeated hand-clapping. The results indicated that these overcorrection procedures were as effective as those that were topographically related to the self-stimulatory behavior.

In a study of R.G. Watters and W.E. Watters (1980), self-stimulatory behavior was effectively reduced by physical exercise. In an earlier study, arm-and-hand exercises were used to eliminate inappropriate hand self-stimulation and later to eliminate foot movements in the same subject (Epstein, Doke, Sajwaj, Sorrell, & Rimmer, 1974). This demonstrated that an overcorrection procedure that is effective for one behavior could be used to reduce the frequency of other (unrelated) behaviors.

Self-injurious behaviors are notoriously difficult to eliminate. They have, for years, been treated with aversives, such as electric shock and corporal punishment (slapping). Recently, however, overcorrection has been demonstrated to be an efficient reducer of self-injurious behavior in subjects for whom other procedures had failed (Horner & Barton, 1980). Freeman, Graham, and Ritvo (1975) reported that nail-picking (to the point of bleeding) in a 6½-year-old child was dramatically reduced by overcorrection. The overcorrection procedure used in this study consisted of holding the child's hands down by her side for one minute each time she engaged in nail-picking. The overcorrection procedure was combined with reinforcement for the subject's appropriate use of her hands. In this study, the positive results were found to be long-lasting.

The head guidance procedure used to eliminate head-weaving (Foxx & Azrin, 1973a), combined with arm exercises, was implemented to reduce head-banging and chin-banging in an eight-year-old retarded boy (Harris & Romanczyk, 1976). This overcorrection procedure was effective in eliminating the self-injurious behavior, and the effects persisted over time.

The generalization of positive effects across settings and over time seems to be dependent upon several factors. Kelly and Drabman (1977) found that the high rate of head-striking behavior of a ten-year-old retarded girl could be reduced by manually raising and lowering the child's arms 20 times, contingent upon each head strike. However, the treatment ultimately failed due to the inability of staff to maintain the treatment. The teachers were unable to continually abandon other students to implement the overcorrection procedure for this one child. In addition, the physical exertion required to guide the child's arms against her resistance proved to be too exhausting for the teachers. The procedure therefore was discontinued, in spite of the initial remarkable results.

Overcorrection procedures have also been effective in treating behaviors other than self-stimulatory behaviors and self-injurious behaviors. Azrin and Foxx (1971) developed a procedure that used "cleanliness training" to overcorrect toilet failures. The cleanliness training was implemented each time the individual urinated in his pants. In this procedure, the individual was immediately given a tepid shower, after which he was required to change his clothes and wash them and to mop the floor or wipe from his chair any traces of his soiling. The toilet-training overcorrection was subsequently developed into a standard procedure for rapidly training retarded individuals (Foxx & Azrin, 1973b).

Azrin and Wesolowski (1975b) demonstrated that overcorrection, or practicing the appropriate behavior, could work where other procedures had failed. Procedures that had failed to reduce floor-sprawling among patients in a residential treatment center included intensive reinforcement for sitting in chairs, making many more chairs available, and continually interrupting instances of floor-sprawling. When the residents were required to practice seating themselves in different chairs for a specified period of time, their floor-sprawling was completely eliminated in eight days.

Foxx (1977) used functional movement training and reinforcement of the appropriate behavior to increase eye contact in three autistic and retarded children. Failure to look at the instructor resulted in a 20-second overcorrection sequence. The children were directed from behind to move their heads in one of three directions: up, down, or straight ahead. The children were given a verbal instruction for each position (for example, "head up"). If a child did not respond within one second, the instructor manually guided the head in the desired direction. If a child began the desired movement at any time during the guidance, the guidance was withdrawn and the instructor used hands to shadow the child's head. The manual guidance was reapplied whenever a child stopped the movement. The children were required to maintain each posture for 15 seconds. When compared with edible and praise reinforcement alone, overcorrection was found to be more effective in producing attending behavior in these children.

TYPES OF OVERCORRECTION

Overcorrection is a procedure designed to counteract the environmental effects of an inappropriate act and to reduce inappropriate responses by requiring the individual to intensively practice "overtly correct forms of relevant behavior" (Foxx & Azrin, 1973a, p. 2). Overcorrection may be classified into two types, according to the inappropriate behavior produced by the individual and the consequent type of practice performed during the overcorrection period. For example, self-stimulatory head-banging may be overcorrected by requiring the individual to practice appropriate head postures. Destructive behavior, such as marking on the walls with crayon, may be overcorrected by requiring the child to clean the marks off the wall and to continue to clean the wall for 20 minutes. Failure to produce a correct response to a learning task, such as turning on the faucet, may be overcorrected by requiring the individual to practice turning on the water 20 times. Inappropriate aggressive behavior, such as spitting, may be overcorrected by using the oral hygiene procedure. All of these examples may be classified as one of two types of overcorrection:

1. *Restitutional overcorrection:* This type of overcorrection requires an individual who has disrupted the environment to put it back the way it was before the disruption occurred. It also requires the disruptor to correct the consequences of the misbehavior by restoring the situation to a state that is much better than that which existed before the disruption (Foxx & Azrin, 1973a). Restitutional overcorrection is a self-correction technique that, by requiring the individual to clean up the messiness that results from the misbehavior, teaches the individual the correct way of acting (Azrin & Wesolowski, 1975a). Its effectiveness suggests that it is reeducative rather than punitive, because the offender learns that behaving in a certain appropriate way is easier than having to overcorrect to a far greater extent than a simple cleanup (Azrin & Wesolowski, 1975a).

2. *Positive practice overcorrection:* This type of overcorrection involves the repeated practice of an appropriate behavior contingent upon the inappropriate behavior (Foxx & Azrin, 1973a). It consists of intensive drilling in correct behaviors. When an individual produces an incorrect behavior or fails to produce a desired response, positive practice overcorrection requires the individual to engage in a repeated exercise that either teaches an alternative (appropriate) behavior or teaches the correct response. Positive practice overcorrection may involve exercises whose features are related to the undesirable behavior but teach a desirable behavior. For example, the overcorrection procedure for self-stimulatory finger-flicking may consist of repeated exercises in putting the hands in the pockets. An overcorrection procedure that teaches a functional skill in the place of an undesirable behavior is preferable, whenever possible. Sometimes, however, it is not possible to devise a positive practice exercise that is topographically related to the inappropriate behavior. In such cases, the repeated practice of an unrelated exercise may be used. Implementation of the overcorrection procedure sometimes requires manual guidance from the instructor. When the desired response is not easily prompted, practicing unrelated exercises serves as a reductive technique for the incorrect behavior or response. Reinforcement of the desired behavior or response then is combined with the unrelated exercises. For

example, it would be difficult manually to prompt eye contact (literally), but the repeated exercise of standing up and sitting down can reduce the "not-looking" behavior. Practicing standing up and sitting down does not, of itself, teach the individual to give eye contact; however, when combined with reinforcement for "looking," it does teach the child to avoid overcorrection by looking at the instructor. Standing up and sitting down is a harmless exercise that, at worst, strengthens leg muscles. Reinforcement of eye contact shows the individual what the expected behavior is.

ADVANTAGES AND DISADVANTAGES

The advantages of overcorrection are considerable in comparison to other reductive or punishment techniques. Overcorrection represents timeout from positive reinforcement because the child does not have the opportunity to be reinforced by the inappropriate behavior; yet it does not have the disadvantages of exclusionary timeout. Exclusionary timeout can give autistic children the opportunity to engage in self-stimulatory behavior, because no one interrupts the behavior. Overcorrection prevents this possibility. In addition, overcorrection prevents the child from engaging in other inappropriate activities, a safeguard that exclusionary timeout does not provide.

Overcorrection is useful in situations where extinction or positive reduction procedures, such as reinforcing incompatible behaviors, have little chance of succeeding. For example, extinction is not useful in situations where self-injurious behavior, if ignored, could result in serious danger to the child. Positive reductive procedures alone generally are not effective with autistic children, particularly when the (self-stimulatory) behaviors are more reinforcing to the child.

The mildly aversive procedures used in overcorrection minimize the negative effects of punishment. The behaviors that are modeled are positive and appropriate, rather than aggressive; thus, the harmful side effects of other punishment procedures are minimized. The overcorrection procedure does not cause emotional anxiety and nervousness, as does physical punishment. The procedure does not involve potential physical harm to the child, nor does it give the child the opportunity to imitate physical aggression.

In overcorrection, adaptive (functional) behaviors are substituted for maladaptive (nonfunctional) ones. The procedure teaches the child acceptable ways of acting through self-correction and new and functional skills through extensive practice. The acquisition of a skill provides the opportunity for reinforcement.

The duration of reinforcement of the inappropriate behavior is brief when overcorrection is used because the behavior is immediately interrupted each time it occurs. Also, practice of the inappropriate behavior is physically prevented by manual guidance. The child is not only prevented from engaging in inappropriate behaviors during the overcorrection procedure, but passive resistance is also prevented because the child is too busy correcting the misbehavior. This requires the child to make an effort to perform correct behaviors. The practice of overcorrection prevents arbitrary usage. That is, the behavior must have occurred for the punishment procedure to be used. Finally, it appears that overcorrection has rapid and long-lasting positive results.

The disadvantages of overcorrection have yet to be fully explored; however, there are a few problems that must be considered. First, it has been noted that the overcorrection procedure can be a physically exhausting and time-consuming procedure. It should not be used with older, combative individuals, since it could develop into a power struggle or an aggressive confrontation. It requires the undivided attention of the teacher and prevents attention to other students in the class. For this reason, teachers who are considering the use of overcorrection must decide if they can afford to leave the other children alone long enough to carry out the procedure; if they cannot, they must enlist the help of aides or other adults. This, as well as the specific type of exercise, requires creativity on the part of the teacher.

Since relatively little research has been done to determine the side effects and the controls necessary for effective overcorrection procedures, the cautions for punishment in general must be remembered.

GUIDELINES

The following procedures will aid in using overcorrection effectively:

- The cleanup practice, or restitutional overcorrection, should be directly related to the misbehavior. The overcorrection should involve cleaning up an area extending beyond the area that was messed up, or it should require an extended period of time.
- The procedure should be consistent; that is, the same procedure should be used each time the inappropriate behavior is observed.
- The procedure should be implemented immediately. The individual should not have the opportunity to be reinforced by the inappropriate behavior, but should be immediately required to practice correct behaviors.

- The instructor should be careful to avoid giving any reinforcement during the overcorrection procedure.
- Although the overcorrection procedure should require physical effort on the part of the child, caution should be taken to avoid overtaxing the very young child. The age and physical condition of the child should always be taken into account.
- Verbal instructions should be given for each exercise. If the child does not respond immediately, the child should be manually guided through the specified activity. The manual guidance should be gradually withdrawn as the child begins to perform the action. If the child stops the movement, manual guidance should be reapplied.
- Emotionality should be avoided.
- Excessive force should be avoided; great care should be taken to ensure that the child is not physically harmed.
- If the child becomes aggressive, the instructor should wait for the aggression to subside. Physical or violent confrontations should be avoided.
- The child's environment should be enriched with reinforcement for alternative appropriate behaviors.

SUMMARY

Punishment procedures, in general, do not teach children appropriate replacement behaviors. Overcorrection, however, is a procedure that, on the one hand, punishes an inappropriate behavior while, on the other hand, teaches an appropriate alternative behavior.

The principle of overcorrection requires the offending individual to engage in repeated practice of an alternative appropriate behavior. If used correctly, overcorrection can be more effective than physical punishment, extinction, or reinforcement of the appropriate behavior alone.

It has been demonstrated that overcorrection is effective in reducing self-stimulatory behavior and self-injury in autistic and severely retarded persons. Also, it has been demonstrated that overcorrection is an effective tool for toilet training, as well as for increasing eye contact in autistic children.

There are two types of overcorrection: (1) restitution and (2) positive practice. Restitutional overcorrection requires an individual who has disrupted the environment to correct the disruption by restoring the situation to a state much better than it was before the upset. Positive practice requires the individual to practice repeatedly an appropriate behavior as a consequence for an inappropriate behavior.

Overcorrection has several advantages. It prevents the individual from engaging in the inappropriate behavior and, at the same time, teaches the individual a new, appropriate behavior as a replacement. It prevents the individual from being reinforced by the inappropriate behavior. It does not involve physical harm to the child.

Disadvantages of overcorrection have not yet been thoroughly investigated; however, the responsible teacher will employ the safeguards used for all forms of punishment.

Chapter 5

Attending

Autistic children generally do not learn from their environment as normal children do (Varmi, Lovaas, Koegel, & Everett, 1979). They often appear to be unconcerned about events around them; they seem distracted by irrelevant sights and sounds, or they seem to close themselves off from anything that could make an impression on them. It has been argued that the resistance to new information or to learning, referred to as "negativism" (Bettelheim, 1967; Morrison et al., 1973), is a device used by autistic children to avoid compliance with adult rules. The idea that negativism is the basis of autistic failure to learn has been disputed (P. Clark & Rutter, 1977). However, teachers and therapists are confronted with autistic behaviors that seem to prevent the acquisition of new and useful information, for whatever reasons. One such behavior is the failure to attend. Attending means, simply, paying attention.

THE IMPORTANCE OF ATTENDING

It can be argued that attention to incoming stimuli or information does not imply processing of that information. In other words, the child who is paying attention may or may not be learning. One may assume, however, that unless the child is able to attend to the task, or attend to environmental stimuli, learning cannot take place. Since actual attending is an internal state, not quantifiable (at this point, anyway) from a behavioral standpoint, the instructor must adapt or create a functional definition of attending. The definition must incorporate those behaviors that, on the face of it, demonstrate that, at the very least, the child is refraining from activity that may interfere with learning or that, at best, the child "appears" to be ready and waiting for some information.[1]

Since autistic children do not attend "naturally," they must be taught to perform those behaviors that, to the best of our knowledge, signify

69

attending. Any teacher who has ever attempted to get autistic children to sit down and pay attention to a task knows that such attempts often end in frustration or disaster. Autistic children do not voluntarily focus their attention on a task (Frankel, Tymchuk, & Simmons, 1976), or they focus too much attention on an insignificant aspect of the task or learning situation (Lovaas et al., 1979). The ability to attend (to pay attention to what is being taught) is crucial in teaching autistic children to communicate or to use language. Unless autistic children can be taught to attend, they cannot transfer the information into short- or long-term memory (McDonald, 1975c). In other words, if nothing relevant gets through, nothing is retained, nothing is learned. In order to teach children to communicate, teachers must be sure that the children are attending to the stimuli being presented.

The importance of teaching autistic children to attend as a first step in the educational process cannot be overstated. Consider the case of a four-year-old autistic boy named David. David darted about the classroom, tipping over flower pots and furniture, rifling shelves and drawers, and clearing table tops of their contents. At every opportunity, David ran out of the school and into the street to peer at automobile engines. He had never spoken to anyone. He had never indicated in any way that he was hungry or thirsty or wanted anything. He never played with other children, and he did not play appropriately with toys. Previous attempts to get him to pay attention by stimulating interest in games or pictures or food met with failure.

A new teacher decided to use a very structured approach with David. The teacher began by teaching him to sit in a chair and pay attention. In less than a month, David could immediately focus his attention on the teacher or on the learning task. He could sit in a chair during an instructional session for a period of 20 minutes. Within two months, he could follow a few simple directions, such as, "stand up" and "come here." One year later, David was able to tell his parents and teachers when he needed to use the toilet, when he wanted something special to eat, or when he wanted a drink of water. He could even say, "Go McDonald's?" At the end of two years, David was placed in a special classroom in his neighborhood school. By then, he could be trusted to function as well as the other children in riding the school bus and in going to and from the playground, cafeteria, and restrooms. Best of all, David could sit at his desk and work on such wondrous tasks as learning to print his name. He had learned by pay attention.

Teaching autistic children to pay attention involves eliminating inappropriate behaviors and building in new, competing behaviors. The principle involved in this process asserts that, if children are attending, they cannot be engaged in inappropriate activities. Inappropriate activities—such as self-stimulation, screaming, running around the classroom, and so on—interfere with the learning process. The purpose of teaching attending is to eliminate the inappropriate activities so that learning can take place (Lovaas, Schreibman, & Koegel, 1974).

Children who have severe behaviors that interfere with attending require stringent, well-planned procedures (Donnellan, 1980; Tanguay, 1976). The plan presented in this chapter is a strict one. It requires that the children learn to give their *full* attention to the instructor. Attending means that the child's whole body is in a position that indicates a readiness to learn. It means that children who are attending are quiet and have their feet on the floor, their hands still, and their eyes on the instructor.

Teaching autistic children to pay attention may take several weeks, or even months, of rigorous training in a one-to-one setting. The length of time it takes depends upon the age of the child, the severity of the disorder, the number of hours per day and days per week spent in training, and the consistency of the training procedures. It is important for professionals working with autistic children to remember that a foundation is being built. Essentially, the time spent in teaching attending is the most valuable of the child's educational career. To cut corners on attending is to build a shaky foundation.

ARRANGING THE ENVIRONMENT

A good teaching session should begin with the careful arrangement of the instructional setting. This must be done *before* the child is brought to the session (unless the instructor is fortunate enough to possess six hands). Everything that is needed for the session should be collected ahead of time and strategically placed. Chairs, table, written program, and so on, should be arranged and assembled. Edible reinforcers and toys should be placed out of reach of the child, since autistic children have been known to appear to have eight arms and legs, well adapted for grabbing and running.

The teaching area should be arranged to minimize distraction that may affect the performance of the child. Some autistic children are easily distracted by colorful wallpaper or upset by background noises, such as music, talking, fire engine sirens, and so on. While a noise-proof chamber is not always possible, or even desirable, the alert instructor will try to free the teaching area from as many obvious distractions as possible.

The attending program begins with the instructor and child sitting in chairs facing each other. Chairs should be placed close enough for the instructor to maintain control of the child. They should be low enough for the child's feet to rest comfortably on the floor, and for the instructor to sit facing the child at eye level. A small desk or table should be placed beside the instructor. The materials needed for the session should be placed on the table.

THE DISCRETE TRIAL FORMAT

The format presented here is the discrete trial format (Donnellan, Gossage, LaVigna, Schuler, & Traphagen, 1977; Koegel, Russo, & Rincover, 1977). Discrete trial means that each trial, or each try, is separate and distinct from the others. The child is given a specified number of trials in which the instructor does or says something to elicit a response from the child. If the response is correct, there is a reward. If the response is incorrect, there is a punishment. A session consists of 10 to 20 trials presented sequentially.

The discrete trial has a distinct beginning and a distinct end; that is, it is possible for everyone to tell when the trial begins and when it ends. It consists of three components: the stimulus, the response, and the consequence.

The Stimulus

The stimulus is anything that stimulates or evokes a particular response from the child (Costello, 1977). It is the signal to which the child must respond. In the attending program, the stimulus is what the instructor says or does. The instructor shows the child how to attend by sitting with feet on the floor and hands on knees and looking at the child. The instructor shows the child how to pay attention by modeling the correct response. To begin the attending program, the instructor also gives the child the direction, "feet down" or "hands still."

It has long been recognized that autistic children require a learning task to be broken down into many small steps and arranged sequentially to complete a larger single task (L. Wing, 1972). This process, known as task analysis, is used in the attending program. The various steps in the attending program are sequenced so that the child learns the easiest task first, with new tasks being added as the child becomes proficient at each previous task. For example, the complete attending task requires the child to sit in a chair with feet on the floor, to keep the hands still, to be quiet, and to look at the instructor. This is quite a bit to expect right off the bat. So the task is broken down into logical units: (1) keeping the feet on the floor, (2) keeping hands still, (3) being quiet, and (4) looking at the instructor. In addition, each unit is broken down into a series of steps that help the child build new behaviors. This is accomplished by prompting, modeling, and prompt fading. The first steps of each unit are designed so that the child is provided lots of help to complete the task (prompting). The child is also shown what to do (modeling). The amount of help is then gradually decreased until the child completes the task without help (prompt fading). At this point, the instructor will find it helpful to remember that the child should not be expected to attend immediately. Attending is what is being taught. It is being shaped gradually, each unit building on the other, to form the complete attending response at the *end* of the program. Concentration on each unit, as it appears in the program, will make the task easier for instructor and child alike.

The Response

The response is what follows the stimulus. It is what the child does or says in response to what has just happened. When a specific stimulus is given, a specific response is expected (Gray & Ryan, 1973). In the example of attending, the stimulus may be, "feet down," and the expected response will be that the child puts feet on the floor and keeps them there. The various steps in the attending program have very specific stimuli and clearly specified responses. Clearly specified responses are necessary in order for the instructor to provide an immediate reaction to the response. The instructor's reaction will either reinforce (increase) the response or punish (decrease) it; therefore, it is imperative that the response be so well-defined that it is immediately recognized as correct or incorrect.

The Consequence

The consequence follows the response. It is how the instructor reacts to the response. Consequences control the direction of the response by either reinforcing it or punishing it. If the response is correct, it should be reinforced. If the response is incorrect, it should be punished.

Consequences should also be planned in advance. The instructor should have an idea of the child's likes and dislikes and have a variety of edibles, toys, games, and so on, that may interest the child. The hope here is that the child will be motivated to work for the reinforcer (Koegel et al., 1980). Likewise, the instructor should have a plan for punishment procedures so that immediate implementation will be possible (Koegel et al., 1977).

THE INTERTRIAL INTERVAL

The delivery of the consequence completes the discrete trial. The next discrete trial begins with the presentation of the next stimulus. The unit of time between the end of one trial and the beginning of the next is called the intertrial interval (Koegel et al., 1977). During this time interval, the data are recorded. If the response given by the child is correct, a plus (+) is recorded during the intertrial interval. If the response given by the child is incorrect, a minus (−) is recorded. An example from the first step of the attending program will illustrate this process. The trial begins with the stimulus, "feet down," given by the instructor. The instructor also gives a prompt by holding the child's feet on the floor for three seconds. The response, given by the child, is compliance with the prompt (the child lets the instructor physically prompt the correct response). This is a correct response. The instructor delivers the consequence, which is, for example, a sip of juice. This ends one discrete trial. The instructor records a plus (+) in the data column of the written program because the child responded correctly. As soon as the plus (+) is recorded (during the intertrial interval), the instructor presents the stimulus for the next trial (Koegel, Dunlap, & Dyer, 1980).

The recording of the data is an essential part of the teaching process (Romanczyk, 1981). Analysis of the percentage of correct responses allows the instructor to make changes in the procedures if the child is not progressing at the expected rate. The analysis of the progress, then, is not based upon guesswork, but upon objective information. At the end of the session (usually after 10 or 20 trials), the instructor should figure the percentage of correct responses by dividing the total number of trials into the number of correct trials.

The following is an example of a recording system that may be used for recording data from discrete trials:

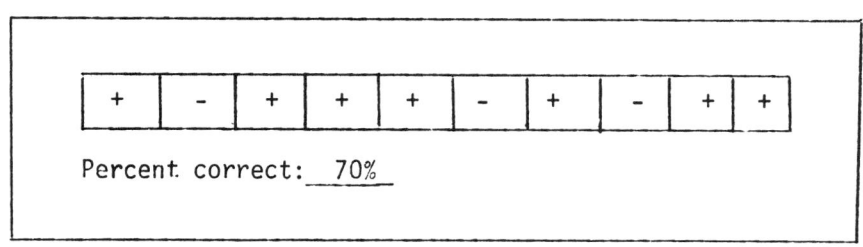

Each square contains information about a discrete trial. It tells whether the child responded correctly or incorrectly. In this example, the child responded correctly on seven of the ten trials. The percentage correct, therefore, was 70 percent. Using this type of information over a period of a few days, the instructor can discern whether or not the child is making progress. If the child consistently obtains low scores, changes in the procedures are necessary. If the child maintains a high score, the instructor continues to use the planned procedures and the child makes the programmed step changes. (An additional form for teacher use in recording data from discrete trials is provided in Appendix B.)

DOCUMENTING THE PROGRAM

All of the information needed to teach the child a new task should be documented in a written program. The written program should include: (1) a statement of the goal, (2) a description of the instructional setting, (3) a list of the materials needed for the session, (4) the criteria for mastery of the program, (5) directions for the delivery of consequences, and (6) the detailed activities. A well-written program will be so explicit that any teacher or therapist could conduct the session.

Statement of the Goal

The statement of the goal should be a simple statement of what the child is expected to accomplish and a time frame for completion. Expected behaviors should be expressed in behavioral terms and should be quantifiable, that is, measurable (Mager, 1975). A goal such as, "The child will sit in a chair and keep feet on the floor for three seconds," is an objective statement of the goal. "The child will behave" is not. The specific behavior to be measured should be stated simply and clearly so that the instructor knows exactly what the end result of the instruction should be. When goals are stated objectively, there is no guesswork involved in measuring the progress toward the completion of the expected goal.

Description of the Setting

The description of the setting should be detailed enough to include special considerations for particular children. For example, Joey may be distracted if he is placed near a window. In such a case, the instructor would include in the description of the setting a suggestion that Joey's sessions be conducted in an enclosed booth away from windows. The description of the setting should also include the arrangement of chairs or other furniture, the position of the instructor and child, and so on.

List of Materials

The list of materials should include everything needed for the session. For the attending program, this will include the written program (instructional procedures), extra data sheets if necessary, a pencil, and a list of items or edibles that will be used for reinforcing correct responses. Other items that might be listed for programs or sessions other than attending are a stop watch, pictures, toys, and objects to be used as stimuli.

Criteria for Mastery

The criteria for mastery are statements of the achievement levels necessary in order for the child to move from one step to the next. They are also indications of the level of correct responses needed to conclude that the child has mastered a complete task (Gray & Ryan, 1973). The criteria for mastery may be stated in percentages, such as, "80 percent correct over 40 trials," or in numbers, such as, "40 consecutive trials completed correctly." The criterion for mastery of the attending program is 80 percent over 40 trials.

Directions for Delivery of Consequences

Directions for the delivery of consequences should explain the procedures for the reinforcement of correct responses and the punishment of incorrect responses. The schedule of reinforcement and punishment should also be stated. For example, reinforcement may be given after every correct response; or it may be better if reinforcement is given after every correct response on Step 1, then after every other correct response on Step 2, and so on, thus fading the reinforcement. The advantage of providing continuous reinforcement (after every correct response) is that the child will more rapidly get into the habit of responding correctly (Smith & Moore, 1966). The same rule applies for punishment. In the attending program, the schedule of reinforcement and punishment is consistent; reinforcement is given after each correct response, and punishment is given after each incorrect response. There are times, however, when the instructor will find it more functional for the child if the frequency of reinforcement is faded (gradually decreased) so that the child does not become dependent upon extrinsic reinforcement.

Activities

The activities should be a detailed step-by-step description of the process for teaching a task. The activities for the discrete trial format are organized into stimulus, response, and consequence categories. The stimulus tells the instructor what to say or do and how to prompt the child. The response specifies what the child is expected to say or do. The consequence tells the instructor how to react to the child's response, whether to reinforce or to punish it.

IMPLEMENTING THE PROGRAM

The attending program breaks the attending task down into four parts corresponding to four separate learning tasks: Part I teaches the child to sit in a chair and keep feet on the floor; Part II teaches the child to keep hands still; Part III teaches the child to be quiet; and Part IV teaches the child to look at the instructor. Each part builds on the previous part so that the child learns the simplest (and easiest to prompt) task first, that is, keeping feet on the floor; then a new behavior is added to the mastered behavior. Thus, the child first learns to keep feet on the floor. Next, the child learns to keep hands still while maintaining the previously mastered behavior of keeping feet on the floor. Next, the child learns to be quiet while maintaining feet on the floor and hands still. Finally, the child learns to look at the instructor while keeping feet on the floor and hands still and being quiet. The task that is mastered by the end of the program is that of sitting quietly in a chair, with feet on the floor and hands still, and looking at the instructor.

Each part is further broken down into five steps. Step 1 incorporates calling the child's name, modeling the desired response, giving a verbal direction, and providing a full prompt. Thus, the instructor says the child's name, shows the child what is expected (models), gives a verbal direction stating the expected behavior, and then physically manipulates the child so that the correct response "position" is tactually perceived by the child. If the child is unable to cognitively comprehend the verbal direction and the model, the full prompt assists the child in performing the task. This step provides the strongest insurance for success for the child, since a correct response requires only that the child cooperate and allow the instructor physically to prompt or guide the correct response.

Step 2 incorporates calling the child's name, modeling, giving a verbal direction, and providing a partial prompt. As in the first step, the instructor says the child's name, models the correct response, and gives a verbal command for the expected behavior. In Step 2, however, the prompt is partial rather than full. The instructor gives a clue or a tactile indication of the expected response by tapping, touching, or partly guiding the part of the child's anatomy involved in the response. Increased responsibility is placed on the child, since the criterion for the correct response is that the child complete the task without further assistance from the instructor.

In Step 3 the instructor calls the child's name, models the correct response, and gives a verbal direction, as in Steps 1 and 2. In Step 3, however, the prompt is omitted. The instructor does not provide physical guidance to help the child complete the task. Rather, the child must perform the task as soon as the verbal direction is given.

Thus far, in Steps 1 through 3, the learning task has proceeded from full prompt, to partial prompt, to no prompt. The instructor's calling of the child's name, presentation of the model, and verbal instruction have remained the same.

In Step 4, the instructor says the child's name and models the response. There is no verbal explanation of the expected response, and there is no prompt. The child is expected to produce the desired behavior that has previously been shaped through prompting and verbal direction.

Step 5 further eliminates the verbal cue by omitting calling the child's name. The instructor simply models the attending behavior. The child must respond by attending, either in part or in entirety, depending upon the specific behavior (Part I, II, III, or IV) being taught.

Suggestions for teaching attending, using this format, have grown out of experience with a number of autistic children of various degrees of severity and intellectual functioning. Generally, the sessions should last no longer than 20 minutes. The discrete trial format is an intense training exercise, which, when rapidly paced, quickly tires the child and the instructor. Several brief sessions, consisting of ten trials each, broken up by short (5 to 15 minutes) periods of free play or other less intense learning activities seem to be the most productive pattern.

The question of how frequently the attending session should be conducted can be answered only by examining the needs of the particular child. Studies have suggested that the more frequent the sessions, the more quickly the child learns (Lovaas, 1968). Certainly, sessions should be conducted at least daily (Zifferblatt, Burton, Horner, & White, 1977) and, wherever possible, several times daily.

Since it has been demonstrated that the most effective teaching situation for autistic children is that in which the instructor works on a one-to-one basis with the child (Israel, 1976), it is strongly suggested that instructors who use the attending program strive to keep this fact in mind. If at all possible, the child should be taught to attend to the instructor on a one-to-one basis first. Later, when the child is attending in all individual sessions and is consistently attending prior to the presentation of new instructional stimuli, the instructor can gradually group children in twos and threes without risking disruptions or without wasting precious educational time. This would be the ideal process. However, we recognize that a teaching ratio of 1:1 is a rare luxury in public schools and in many teaching centers. Therefore, if the teacher or instructor can provide, at the minimum, one hour of individual attending instruction per day, this will greatly enhance the autistic child's chances of remaining in the classroom and eventually being able to function in groups of several children.

To illustrate more clearly the design and content of the attending program, Appendix 5–A presents detailed instructions for establishing the program's goals and setting and for providing the requisite materials, criteria, consequences, and activities. Activities for each part (I–IV) and its five component steps are shown in Table 5A–1. (An additional program form for teacher use is provided in Appendix C.)

SUMMARY

The ability to pay attention is an essential prerequisite for learning. The purpose of teaching autistic children to pay attention is to eliminate inappropriate competing behaviors so that learning can take place. Attending is defined as sitting quietly in a chair, with feet and hands down and eyes on the instructor or learning materials.

The teaching of attending begins with the careful arrangement of the teaching environment. The physical setting is arranged so that unwanted distractions are prevented and necessary materials are easily accessible. The discrete trial format—consisting of stimulus, response, and consequence—is used to teach attending. The stimulus is recognized as what the instructor says or does to elicit a particular response from the child. The response is what the child says or does following the stimulus. The response is either correct or incorrect. The consequence is what the instructor does to either reinforce or punish the response. The unit of time between the end of one trial and the beginning of the next is called the intertrial interval. This time is used to record the data (an essential component of discrete trial teaching).

The task of teaching the child to attend is broken down into carefully sequenced steps that employ prompting, modeling, and prompt fading.

NOTE

1. There is disagreement among professionals regarding the nature of attending and the role of attention as a prerequisite for learning. Until evidence to the contrary is demonstrated, we will assume that attending can be defined in behavioral terms and can, thus, be measured as such. No inference is made that attending means learning or that what we are measuring is the actual physiological process of attending.

Appendix 5–A

Instructions and Format for Implementing an Attending Program

INSTRUCTIONS FOR ATTENDING

Goal

- Part I—The child will sit in a chair with both feet on the floor.
- Part II—The child will sit in a chair with both feet on the floor and hands still.
- Part III—The child will sit in a chair with both feet on the floor and hands still and will be quiet.
- Part IV—The child will sit in a chair with both feet on the floor and hands still, will be quiet, and will look at the instructor.
- Expected completion: _____(filled in by the instructor).

Setting

All sessions will take place in the classroom, in an enclosed booth. Two small chairs should be placed facing each other. A small table should be placed next to the instructor's chair. All materials should be placed on the table. Edible reinforcers should be placed out of the reach of the child. The session will be conducted from _____until _____(filled in by the instructor) daily.

Materials

Two small chairs, a small table, the written program, extra data sheets, a pencil, and reinforcers (orange juice and bits of graham cracker, for example): _____(filled in by the instructor).

Criterion for Mastery

Eighty percent correct in 40 trials.

Procedures for the Delivery of Consequences

Reinforcement

Following each correct response, the instructor gives the child social reinforcement, such as, "Good! Your feet are on the floor," and a backup reinforcement, such as juice or a bit of cracker.

Punishment

Following each incorrect response, the instructor implements overcorrection as follows:

- Part I: A correct response requires that the child keep feet on the floor for three seconds. If the child responds incorrectly by failing to keep feet on the floor:
    1. In a firm voice, say, "Feet down."
    2. Grasp the child's feet and place them on the floor.
    3. Hold the child's feet down for two to three seconds.
    4. Repeat the exercise ten times in succession.

- Part II: A correct response requires that the child keep feet on the floor and hands still for three seconds. If the child responds incorrectly by failing to keep hands still:
    1. In a firm voice, say, "Hands still."
    2. Grasp the child's hands and place them on the child's knees.
    3. Hold the child's hands down for two to three seconds.
    4. Repeat the exercise ten times in succession.

- Part III: A correct response requires that the child keep feet on the floor and hands still and be quiet for three seconds. If the child responds incorrectly by failing to be quiet:
    1. In a firm voice, say, "You're not quiet. Stand up."
    2. Grasp the child by the shoulders and guide to standing position.
    3. In a firm voice, say, "Sit down."
    4. Grasp the child by the shoulders and guide to sitting position.
    5. Repeat the exercise ten times in succession.

- Part IV: A correct response requires that the child keep feet on the floor and hands still and be quiet and look at the instructor for three seconds. If the child responds incorrectly by failing to look at the instructor:

1. In a firm voice, say, "You're not looking. Stand up."
2. Grasp the child by the shoulders and guide to standing position.
3. In a firm voice, say, "Sit down."
4. Grasp the child by the shoulders and guide to sitting position.
5. Repeat the exercise ten times in succession.

Activities

Activities for each part (I–IV) and its five component steps in the attending program are listed in Table 5A–1.

Table 5A–1 Component Activities of an Attending Program

ATTENDING PART I
Step 1

Stimulus	Prompt	Response	Consequence	Data
1. Instructor says, "(child's name)."				Session 1: Date ____
2. Instructor models attending by sitting with feet on floor, hands on knees, and looking at child.				% Correct ____
3. Instructor says, "Feet down."				Session 2: Date ____
	4. Instructor grasps child's feet, places them on the floor, and holds them in place for three seconds.			% Correct ____
		5. Child keeps both feet on the floor without resisting.		Session 3: Date ____
			6. Instructor delivers social and backup reinforcement.	% Correct ____
		7. Child resists prompt; does not keep feet on the floor.		Session 4: Date ____
			8. Instructor implements overcorrection.	% Correct ____

Table 5A–1 continued

ATTENDING PART I
Step 2

Stimulus	Prompt	Response	Consequence	Data
1. Instructor says, "(child's name)."				Session 1: Date _____ % Correct _____
2. Instructor models attending by sitting with feet on floor, hands on knees, and looking at child.				
3. Instructor says, "Feet down."				Session 2: Date _____ % Correct _____
	4. Instructor touches child's feet, then points to floor.			
		5. Child puts both feet on floor and keeps them there for three seconds.		Session 3: Date _____ % Correct _____
			6. Instructor delivers social and backup reinforcement.	
		7. Child does not put feet on floor, or does not keep them there for three seconds.		Session 4: Date _____ % Correct _____
			8. Instructor implements overcorrection.	

ATTENDING PART I
Step 3

			Session 1: Date _____
1. Instructor says, "(child's name)."			
			% Correct _____
2. Instructor models attending by sitting with feet on floor, hands on knees, and looking at child.			Session 2: Date _____
			% Correct _____
3. Instructor says, "Feet down."	4. Child puts both feet on floor and keeps them there for three seconds.		Session 3: Date _____
		5. Instructor delivers social and backup reinforcement.	% Correct _____
	6. Child does not put feet on floor, or does not keep them there for three seconds.		Session 4: Date _____
		7. Instructor implements overcorrection.	% Correct _____

Table 5A–1 continued

ATTENDING PART I
Step 4

Stimulus	Prompt	Response	Consequence	Data
1. Instructor says, "(child's name)."				Session 1: Date___ % Correct___
2. Instructor models attending by sitting with feet on floor, hands on knees, and looking at child.				Session 2: Date___ % Correct___
		3. Child puts both feet on floor and keeps them there for three seconds.		Session 3: Date___ % Correct___
			4. Instructor delivers social and backup reinforcement.	
		5. Child does not put feet on floor, or does not keep them there for three seconds.		Session 4: Date___ % Correct___
			6. Instructor implements overcorrection.	

ATTENDING PART I
Step 5

		Session 1: ___
		Date ___
1. Instructor models attending by sitting with feet on floor, hands on knees, and looking at child.		% Correct ___
	2. Child puts both feet on floor and keeps them there for three seconds.	Session 2: ___
		Date ___
		3. Instructor delivers social and backup reinforcement.
		% Correct ___
		Session 3: ___
		Date ___
	4. Child does not put feet on floor, or does not keep them there for three seconds.	% Correct ___
		5. Instructor implements overcorrection.
		Session 4: ___
		Date ___
		% Correct ___

Table 5A–1 continued

ATTENDING PART II
Step 1

Stimulus	Prompt	Response	Consequence	Data
1. Instructor says, "(child's name)."				Session 1: Date _____ [grid] % Correct _____
2. Instructor models attending by sitting with feet on floor, hands on knees, and looking at child.				Session 2: Date _____ [grid] % Correct _____
3. Instructor says, "Feet down, hands still."	4. Instructor grasps child's hands, places them on child's knees, and holds them in place for three seconds.	5. Child puts both feet on floor and keeps hands on knees without resisting.	6. Instructor delivers social and backup reinforcement.	Session 3: Date _____ [grid] % Correct _____
		7. Child resists prompt, or does not put feet on floor.	8. Instructor implements overcorrection.	Session 4: Date _____ [grid] % Correct _____

ATTENDING PART II
Step 2

Step	Session 1: Date ___	Session 2: Date ___	Session 3: Date ___	Session 4: Date ___
1. Instructor says, "(child's name)."				
2. Instructor models attending by sitting with feet on floor, hands on knees, and looking at child.				
3. Instructor says, "Feet down, hands still."				
4. Instructor touches child's hands and points to child's knees.				
5. Child puts both feet on floor, puts hands down, and keeps them there for three seconds.				
6. Instructor delivers social and backup reinforcement.				
7. Child does not keep feet on floor and hands still for three seconds.				
8. Instructor implements overcorrection.				
% Correct	___	___	___	___

Table 5A–1 continued

ATTENDING PART II
Step 3

Stimulus	Prompt	Response	Consequence	Data
1. Instructor says, "(child's name)."				Session 1: Date____
				% Correct____
2. Instructor models attending by sitting with feet on floor, hands on knees, and looking at child.				Session 2: Date____
				% Correct____
3. Instructor says, "Feet down, hands still."				Session 3: Date____
		4. Child puts both feet on floor, puts hands down, and keeps them there for three seconds.		% Correct____
			5. Instructor delivers social and backup reinforcement.	Session 4: Date____
		6. Child does not keep feet on floor and hands still for three seconds.		% Correct____
			7. Instructor implements overcorrection.	

ATTENDING PART II
Step 4

	Session 1: Date ____ % Correct ____	Session 2: Date ____ % Correct ____	Session 3: Date ____ % Correct ____	Session 4: Date ____ % Correct ____
1. Instructor says, "(child's name)."				
2. Instructor models attending by sitting with feet on floor, hands on knees, and looking at child.				
3. Child puts both feet on floor, puts hands down, and keeps them there for three seconds.				
4. Instructor delivers social and backup reinforcement.				
5. Child does not put feet on floor and hands still for three seconds.				
6. Instructor implements overcorrection.				

Table 5A–1 continued

ATTENDING PART II
Step 5

Stimulus	Prompt	Response	Consequence	Data
1. Instructor models attending by sitting with feet on floor, hands on knees, and looking at child.				Session 1: Date ____ % Correct ____
		2. Child puts both feet on floor, puts hands down, and keeps them there for three seconds.		Session 2: Date ____ % Correct ____
			3. Instructor delivers social and backup reinforcement.	Session 3: Date ____ % Correct ____
		4. Child does not keep feet on floor and hands still for three seconds.		Session 4: Date ____ % Correct ____
			5. Instructor implements overcorrection.	

ATTENDING PART III
Step 1

Step		Session 1: Date ___ % Correct ___
1. Instructor says, "(child's name)."		
2. Instructor models attending by sitting with feet on floor, hands on knees and looking at child.		
3. Instructor says, "Feet down, hands still, be quiet."		Session 2: Date ___ % Correct ___
4. Instructor holds index finger on child's lips for three seconds.		
	5. Child puts both feet on floor, puts hands down and is quiet for three seconds.	Session 3: Date ___ % Correct ___
		6. Instructor delivers social and backup reinforcement.
	7. Child resists prompt or does not keep feet on floor and hands still for three seconds.	Session 4: Date ___ % Correct ___
		8. Instructor implements overcorrection.

Table 5A–1 continued

ATTENDING PART III
Step 2

Stimulus	Prompt	Response	Consequence	Data
1. Instructor says, "(child's name)."				Session 1: Date _____ % Correct _____
2. Instructor models attending by sitting with feet on floor, hands on knees, and looking at child.				
3. Instructor says, "Feet down, hands still, be quiet."				Session 2: Date _____ % Correct _____
	4. Instructor holds index finger a few inches away from child's lips.			
		5. Child puts feet on floor, puts hands down, and is quiet for three seconds.		Session 3: Date _____ % Correct _____
			6. Instructor delivers social and backup reinforcement.	
		7. Child does not keep feet on floor with hands still and is not quiet for three seconds.		Session 4: Date _____ % Correct _____
			8. Instructor implements overcorrection.	

ATTENDING PART III
Step 3

			Session 1: ___ Date ___ % Correct ___	Session 2: ___ Date ___ % Correct ___	Session 3: ___ Date ___ % Correct ___	Session 4: ___ Date ___ % Correct ___
1. Instructor says, "(child's name)."						
2. Instructor models attending by sitting with feet on floor, hands on knees, and looking at child.						
3. Instructor says, "Feet down, hands still, be quiet."						
	4. Child puts both feet on floor, puts hands down, and is quiet for three seconds.					
		5. Instructor delivers social and backup reinforcement.				
	6. Child does not keep feet on floor with hands still and is not quiet for three seconds.					
		7. Instructor implements overcorrection.				

Table 5A–1 continued

ATTENDING PART III
Step 4

Stimulus	Prompt	Response	Consequence	Data
1. Instructor says, "(child's name)."				Session 1: Date _____ % Correct _____
2. Instructor models attending by sitting with feet on floor, hands on knees, and looking at child.				Session 2: Date _____ % Correct _____
		3. Child puts both feet on floor, puts hands down, and is quiet for three seconds.		Session 3: Date _____ % Correct _____
			4. Instructor delivers social and backup reinforcement.	
		5. Child does not keep feet on floor with hands still and is not quiet for three seconds.		Session 4: Date _____ % Correct _____
			6. Instructor implements overcorrection.	

ATTENDING PART III
Step 5

			Session 1: Date _____ <table><tr><td></td><td></td></tr><tr><td></td><td></td></tr></table>% Correct _____
1. Instructor models attending by sitting with feet on floor, hands on knees, and looking at child.			
	2. Child puts both feet on floor, puts hands down, and is quiet for three seconds.		Session 2: Date _____ % Correct _____
		3. Instructor delivers social and backup reinforcement.	Session 3: Date _____ % Correct _____
	4. Child does not keep feet on floor with hands still and is not quiet for three seconds.		Session 4: Date _____ % Correct _____
		5. Instructor implements overcorrection.	

Table 5A–1 continued

ATTENDING PART IV
Step 1

Stimulus	Prompt	Response	Consequence	Data
1. Instructor says, "(child's name)."				Session 1: Date _____ % Correct _____
2. Instructor models attending by sitting with feet on floor, hands on knees, and looking at child.				Session 2: Date _____ % Correct _____
3. Instructor says, "Feet down, hands still, be quiet and look at me."	4. Instructor holds edible in front of eyes and holds child's face to focus attention on edible for three seconds.	5. Child puts both feet on floor, puts hands down, is quiet, and looks for three seconds.		Session 3: Date _____ % Correct _____
		7. Child resists prompt or does not keep feet on floor and hands still and is not quiet for three seconds.	6. Instructor delivers social and backup reinforcement.	Session 4: Date _____ % Correct _____
			8. Instructor implements overcorrection.	

ATTENDING PART IV
Step 2

Step	Session 1: Date _____ % Correct _____	Session 2: Date _____ % Correct _____	Session 3: Date _____ % Correct _____	Session 4: Date _____ % Correct _____
1. Instructor says, "(child's name)."				
2. Instructor models attending by sitting with feet on floor, hands on knees, and looking at child.				
3. Instructor says, "Feet down, hands still, be quiet and look at me."				
4. Instructor holds edible in front of eyes.				
5. Child puts both feet on floor, puts hands down, is quiet and looks for three seconds.				
6. Instructor delivers social and backup reinforcement.				
7. Child does not keep feet on floor with hands still, is not quiet, and does not look for three seconds.				
8. Instructor implements overcorrection.				

Table 5A–1 continued

ATTENDING PART IV
Step 3

Stimulus	Prompt	Response	Consequence	Data
1. Instructor says, "(child's name)."				Session 1: Date _____ % Correct _____
2. Instructor models attending by sitting with feet on floor, hands on knees, and looking at child.				
3. Instructor says, "Feet down, hands still, be quiet and look at me."				Session 2: Date _____ % Correct _____
		4. Child puts both feet on floor, puts hands down, is quiet and looks for three seconds.		
			5. Instructor delivers social and backup reinforcement.	Session 3: Date _____ % Correct _____
		6. Child does not keep feet on floor with hands still, is not quiet, and does not look for three seconds.		
			7. Instructor implements overcorrection.	Session 4: Date _____ % Correct _____

ATTENDING PART IV
Step 4

	Session 1: Date _____	Session 2: Date _____	Session 3: Date _____	Session 4: Date _____
1. Instructor says, "(child's name)."				
2. Instructor models attending by sitting with feet on floor, hands on knees, and looking at child.				
3. Child puts both feet on floor, puts hands down, is quiet, and looks for three seconds.				
4. Instructor delivers social and backup reinforcement.				
5. Child does not keep feet on floor with hands still, is not quiet, and does not look for three seconds.				
6. Instructor implements overcorrection.				
% Correct _____				

Table 5A–1 continued

ATTENDING PART IV
Step 5

Stimulus	Prompt.	Response	Consequence	Data
1. Instructor models attending by sitting with feet on floor, hands on knees, and looking at child.				Session 1: Date _____ % Correct _____
		2. Child puts both feet on floor, puts hands down, is quiet, and looks for three seconds.		Session 2: Date _____ % Correct _____
			3. Instructor delivers social and backup reinforcement.	Session 3: Date _____ % Correct _____
		4. Child does not keep feet on floor with hands still, is not quiet, and does not look for three seconds.		Session 4: Date _____ % Correct _____
			5. Instructor implements overcorrection.	

Chapter 6

Approaches to Teaching Communication

SPEECH, LANGUAGE, AND COMMUNICATION

The terms *language, speech,* and *communication* are frequently used interchangeably; however, they are not synonymous (Dale, 1972). Language is a tool that is used to communicate (Langacker, 1967), but it is not the same as communication. Language is a system of rules used by a community (for example, the community of speakers of English) to express ideas or concepts. It is a symbolic system. The use of language involves cognitive abilities that help individuals to organize and categorize information that their senses convey to them.

Speech is a manifestation of language (Moores, 1981). It is behavior (Slobin, 1971), that is, the vocal behavior that carries the linguistic message.

There are many forms or modes of expressing language. Speech is one mode of expression. Written language and manual sign language are also modes of expressing language. Communication modes involve a physical or outward form for conveying ideas. Therefore, speech, as an expressive mode, is the verbal form for expressing language.

Communication refers to the establishment of a relationship. The term is derived from the Latin root *communicatio,* which means sharing or distributing (MacKay, 1972). Thus, communication involves two participants: a sender and a receiver. The term also implies that, through communication, there is an effect upon the recipient of the message. Communication is a process of exchange between the initiator and the receiver. In other words, two people who are communicating are engaging in the act of sharing information. When the initiator (the sender of the message) shares some information with the receiver, the receiver is affected in some way. For example, the young infant cries, signifying some distress (hunger, thirst, pain, messy diapers, and so on). The mother receives the message and takes action to relieve her infant's discomfort. This illustrates the functional role of communication.

There are, of course, rules that govern the use of communication. To be able to communicate is to be able to understand and use those unwritten laws that allow individuals of a given community or society to engage meaningfully in a shared event (Lucas, 1980). Severely handicapped children must begin instruction with the establishment of the function of communication before complex language can begin to be realized (Sailor, Guess, Goetz, Schuler, Utley, & Baldwin, 1980).

Language and speech involve a highly developed and complex system of rules. Semantic rules (rules for meaning), syntactic rules (rules for structure), and pragmatic rules (rules for meaning in context) govern the use of language; and phonological rules (rules for combining sounds) govern speech. Communication, however, can take place in the absence of linguistic rules. Communication involves rules, but these rules are less complex, perhaps more primitive. Bodily contact is an example of a nonverbal (nonlinguistic) signal (Argyle, 1972). Hitting and pushing are acts that communicate aggression. On the other hand, hugging, kissing, and shaking hands can communicate affection or greetings.

Though every community of humans has developed spoken language (Lyons, 1972), and speech is the preferred mode of communication, communication can occur without language or speech. This distinction is important in the assessment of handicapped children and in the development of communication and language programs.

Nonspeech communication occurs daily among individuals. Smiling, frowning, waving, standing close, and folding the arms across the chest are examples of natural communicative gestures used to convey messages. Generally, communicative gestures are used to supplement or add information to verbal (spoken) language. However, when the speech or language systems break down or fail to develop, alternative communication systems may be devised to aid the individual. Such manufactured communication systems, to be functional, must assist the individual in establishing a relationship with others in the environment. In the following sections we examine the design and implementation of alternative communication systems for use with autistic children.

ASSESSING COMMUNICATIVE BEHAVIOR

Autistic children are typically uncommunicative; that is, they fail to establish a "sharing" relationship with others. Some autistic children possess speech and the ability to use language, yet they fail to communicate. Others are nonverbal; that is, they do not use language or speech. Nor have they developed an alternative, acceptable means of communication. Tantrums may express distress or dissatisfaction, but tantrums are not an acceptable form of communication. Some autistic children emit vocal sounds, or they may spout strings of words, but these forms of vocal behavior are generally not used for communicative purposes. They are not intended to establish relationships with other individuals.

Standardized testing procedures may be used to evaluate the speech and language behavior of autistic children. Syntactic, semantic, pragmatic, and phonological aspects of verbal behavior can be evaluated by means of formal testing or observation. (The purpose here is not to critique existing standardized language tests, but rather to provide the educator or therapist with means for evaluating communicative behavior. See J. Miller, 1981, and Thorum, 1981, for comprehensive lists of standardized tests of linguistic ability.)

Prerequisites for most formal testing procedures require that the child have some forms of verbal expression. In the present context, we shall deal with procedures for evaluating the communicative behavior of the nonverbal child.

Assessment procedures for nonverbal children are generally informal and require several periods of observation in a variety of settings. Even verbal, echolalic children require close observation to determine whether or not communication is present.

Assessment of communicative behavior should be concerned with identifying underlying language skills and purposeful attempts to engage others in some reciprocal event. Evaluation involves defining those skills or abilities that the child clearly exhibits and those that the child needs to learn. The goal or end result of the evaluation should be a profile of the child that enables the instructor to develop a plan for sequencing the skills to be taught.

Lord and O'Neill (1980) have developed a four-step model for prescriptive evaluation, that is, evaluation that leads to programming. The model includes (1) a list of the child's strengths and weaknesses, including what the child can do in the best of circumstances as well as what the child cannot reliably do; (2) structured observation in the child's own environment to determine consistent behaviors and environmental effects on the child's behavior; (3) a needs assessment to outline current and long-term goals for the child; and (4) a list of activities and strategies to help the child achieve the goals. This model provides a useful system for analyzing and planning communication programs for autistic children.

The examination of strengths and weaknesses must include an assessment of prerequisite behaviors that indicate that the child is "ready" for a communication program. These behaviors include the ability to attend to the instructor or to instructional stimuli, the elimination of self-stimulatory behavior, and the ability to imitate motor movements (Flaharty, 1976; Stremel & Waryas, 1974). Self-stimulation and nonattending interfere with learning. Failure to imitate indicates an absence of the cognitive associations necessary for the child to connect a symbol with its associated meaning (Flaharty, 1976). These "readiness" behaviors will have to be taught before the child can begin to learn to communicate.

The quality of communicative behavior may be assessed by observing the child's responses to the environment. Such responses indicate the child's capacity to receive and process information, which will ultimately determine the child's potential for communicative ability (Sanders, 1976). Involvement with objects rather than people, lack of eye contact, lack of responses to the human voice, lack of social smiling, and lack of gestural means to indicate needs and desires are all signs of failure to communicate on a very basic social level. Behaviors that are communicative include showing objects or pictures to others, looking at others, pointing, gesturing, offering objects to adults, offering but not releasing objects, and giving on request (Kiernan, 1981). The evaluator should note whether or not the child explores the environment; shows an interest in, listens to, or responds to vocalizations; vocalizes (other than to make distress sounds or vocal self-stimulation); or attempts to imitate. Failure in any of these areas indicates a deficit in prerequisite communication skills (Uzgiris & Hunt, 1975).

The determination of a child's potential for developing spoken language is tenuous at best (Shane, 1981). However, an assessment of communicative ability must include an assessment of potential. Potential for communication, in the broadest sense, means determining whether or not the child will be able to use some simple form of communication to express needs and desires. The establishment of a communicative system means that the child must be taught that communicative efforts can have an impact. When the environment responds to the child's communicative efforts, a social relationship is established (Lucas, 1980). Real communication occurs when the child uses the communication system to interact spontaneously with others. The use of a simple form of communication to express basic needs and desires will be the ultimate goal for many nonverbal autistic children.

Determining the potential for language involves assessing the child's capacity for learning to use a complex system of rules for interacting with others. The course of language or communication development will depend upon the child's potential for language and speech usage.

There are some guidelines that can help the instructor determine if a program for speech development should be designed or if an alternative mode of communication should be planned for the child. On a physiological level, control of the speech musculature can be inferred from the child's ability to eat and drink. The potential for sound production can be assumed if vocal noises are consistently produced by the child. Of course, the speech mechanism may be intact but sound production may still be random or self-stimulatory. In order to use speech, the nonverbal child must be able to imitate. Whether or not the child can be taught to imitate sounds and words can be determined, to some degree, by whether or not the child can learn to imitate motor movements. If the child can imitate motor movements but fails to imitate speech, an alternative communication system, such as manual communication (discussed later in this chapter), may be useful.

Assessment of communicative functioning should include a complete audiological and visual examination. Symptoms of hearing or visual deficits are often disguised as behavioral or cognitive disorders. It is essential that medical deficits be ruled out or corrected before beginning instruction. Obviously, physical impairments can interfere with learning. Valuable educational time is wasted when therapists assume that failure to learn must be a function of a behavioral or cognitive deficit. Thus, a thorough educational evaluation must not be limited to particular aspects of the child's behavior; it must encompass all areas that provide information about the child as a whole being.

STAGES IN DEVELOPING COMMUNICATION PROGRAMS

Relevant Factors

A communication program should begin with a simple, functional curriculum. In order to be functional, the communication system must give the child something to "talk" about and must elicit a response from others (Ruder & Smith, 1974). Instructional objectives should be defined in terms of critical functions (White, 1980).

Several factors must be considered in deciding which aspects of communication are *critical, essential,* and *useful* for the child. The efficiency and effectiveness of the initial vocabulary must be considered. In other words, will the child be able to use the words frequently? Will the vocabulary produce the desired communicative effect? For example, teaching the child to say "food" has a useful purpose; the child gains physical satisfaction from the acquisition of food and also gains communicative competence by eliciting the desired response from others. The satisfaction of physical needs is a critical function for the child. On the other hand, learning to place round pegs into round holes is not critical to the severely handicapped child who has no communicative ability.

The child's current and future environment must also be considered. Will others in the environment encourage the child to use the communication system? Will significant adults and/or siblings respond to the child's communicative attempts? Will they learn to use the child's communicative system themselves? Answers to these questions will determine which type of communication system is best suited to the child's needs and the extent to which it should be developed.

Many children require thousands of trials to acquire a skill, and many fail to use acquired skills in settings other than the training setting (Goetz, Schuler, & Sailor, 1979). It is important, therefore, to select simple communicative goals that will be useful for the child and that are likely to occur consistently in the child's environment. It is also important to train the child in various locations so that generalization will be facilitated (Handleman, 1981; Handleman & Harris, 1980; Harris, 1975).

In selecting an initial vocabulary, function for the child should be paramount. The child should experience the ability to manipulate the environment by communication. Carlson (1981) has provided a list of sources from which an initial vocabulary can be derived. Parents and other family members can provide information about the child's likes and dislikes. Parents can be asked to indicate where the child spends a lot of time, and a list of preferred items in that setting can constitute an initial vocabulary. Parents or caretakers should also be asked to provide lists of words and activities that are common in the child's environment.

The communication program should be based on realistic goals for the child. The goals must take into consideration the expectations for communicative behavior, the kinds of interaction that normally take place between the child and others in the environment, how the communication system can help the child become an active participant in social interaction, and what is the best, most systematic approach for teaching desirable and appropriate communication (J.F. Miller & Yoder, 1974).

Finally, it is critical to begin communication instruction with strict training procedures. Shaping, prompting, prompt fading, and chaining can be incorporated into direct instructional techniques (Kysela, Hillyard, McDonald, & Ahlsten-Taylor, 1981). The most effective procedures are those that present an ordered series of steps, each one to be accomplished before taking the next one (Premack, 1970).

Imitation Training

Imitation training is the first step in teaching autistic children to communicate. In recent years there has been a great deal of discussion about the function of imitation in teaching language to nonverbal children (J.A. Courtright & I.C. Courtright, 1979). Educators disagree on the merits of imitation training; objections are generally based on what is known about the role of imitation in normal language development. However, communication programs for nonverbal children need not be based on developmental data.

Communication programs that base initial language development on imitation have demonstrated that imitation is an important first step (Gray & Ryan, 1973; Kent, 1974; Lovaas, 1968; Murdock & Hartmann, 1975; Striefel, 1974). For many autistic children, imitation provides a vehicle for responding or interacting for the first time (M.L. Cole & J.T. Cole, 1981). While imitation may not be necessary for normal language acquisition (N.S. Rees, 1975), it is a useful tool in remediation (D. Baer, Peterson, & Sherman, 1967; W.A. Bricker & D.D. Bricker, 1974). Children who can be taught to imitate motor responses are more likely to learn to use some form of communication. Children who can be taught to imitate speech are more likely to learn to use language (Guess, Sailor, & D.M. Baer, 1974; Lovaas, 1977).

Initial Steps

Imitation training should begin with training the child to imitate nonverbal (motor) movements. Imitation of simple movements that involve the large muscles of the body, such as raising the arms, should be taught first; then the finer, less distinct movements—such as smiling, frowning, and other facial expressions—should be taught (Lovaas, 1981). The purpose of teaching autistic children to imitate is to direct attention to a required response to a specific request or action. Ultimately, imitation is used to establish verbal control over the child's nonverbal behaviors (Lovaas, 1981).

Autistic children typically do not imitate (Carr, 1976). Therefore, a systematic procedure for teaching imitation is necessary. This procedure begins with physically prompting the complete behavior modeled by the adult. On subsequent trials, the amount of physical guidance is gradually decreased until the child's response models the adult's behavior (Striefel & Owens, 1980).

Imitation training begins with motor imitation because motor imitation is important in establishing response during instruction, even though it may not generalize to vocal imitation (Goetz et al., 1979; Guess et al., 1974). Imitation of motor movements should begin with large or gross motor activities. Large body movements—such as standing up, raising the arms, or jumping up and down—are simple. They involve the use of larger, less complex muscle control. Simple motor movements are more easily distinguished than more subtle motor movements. Also, gross motor movements are more easily manipulated by the instructor. This is important in the early stages of imitation, when prompting and shaping are used to establish a response.

Imitation of gross motor movements should be followed by imitation of fine motor movements. Fine motor movements include pointing, touching objects, pointing to body parts, smiling, frowning, and using other facial expressions. A carefully designed imitation program will lead the child from imitating gross motor movements to imitating fine motor movements, which ultimately involve the lips, tongue, and other oral structures (Sloane, Johnston, & Harris, 1968).

The next step in imitation training is to teach the child to imitate sounds. By this time, the child should be producing nonverbal imitative responses and should understand that imitation is the expected response. Since intentional sound production is quite a complex task, however, the child may not possess the capacity to control sound output, even though motor imitation may now be an established response. In such cases, an alternative communication mode, such as manual signing, may be desirable.

Implementing the Program

The following program may be used to establish imitative behavior in autistic children. The program consists of three steps: Step 1 uses the full physical prompt to guide manually the child's response; Step 2 uses the partial prompt; and Step 3 uses no prompt. Step 2 may be broken down into a series of substeps that gradually fade the amount of physical guidance given to the child. For example, in teaching a child to imitate raising the arms, the system of substep prompts in Step 2 could be implemented as follows:

- The instructor raises the child's arms, then releases the hold on the child's arms.
- The instructor raises the child's arms halfway, then releases the hold.
- The instructor touches the child's wrists, then points to the space where the child's arms should be (above the head).
- The instructor touches the child's wrists.
- The instructor points to the child's wrists.

Prompts can be faded in many ways. The key to successful prompt fading is to begin by providing the child with enough manual guidance to ensure consistent success; then the amount of guidance is gradually and systematically decreased. The gradual, step-by-step decrease helps to prevent the child from becoming dependent upon the prompt. Appendix 6–A presents detailed instructions for establishing an imitation program's goals and setting and/or providing the requisite materials, criteria, consequences, and activities. Activities for each of the three steps in establishing imitative behavior in a child are shown in Table 6A–1. (An additional program form for teacher use is provided in Appendix C.)

DEVELOPING COMMUNICATION PROGRAMS FOR THE NONVERBAL CHILD

In recent years, attention has been focused on methods of instructing the severely retarded or nonverbal autistic child. Several types of communication systems have evolved to assist handicapped individuals in learning to use language. Gestural communication modes include systems that involve bodily movements and require no instrumentation. Examples of gestural modes are American sign language, signing exact English, and pointing (Silverman, 1980). Gestural modes have recently been used successfully with nonverbal autistic children. This is discussed in the following section. Other types of nonspeech communication systems are examined briefly below. (For more detailed explanations of nonspeech communication systems and their use, see M. Cohen, 1979, and Silverman, 1980.)

Types of Nonspeech Communication Systems

Most nonspeech communication programs are designed to teach functional responses rather than elaborate grammatical structures. One such system is the Non-Speech Language Initiation Program (Non-SLIP) (Carrier & Peak, 1975). Non-SLIP involves the use of color-coded plastic symbols to teach rules of communication. It is intended to be an initial program for teaching children the process for learning communication skills. Its goals include organization of environmental events, organization of responses to the environment, and a mode of communication that does not require spoken words. The objective is to help children sort and simplify the communicative process so that initial communication can take place. The Non-SLIP training program prepares the child for future instruction in more traditional forms of communication. Rather than adhering to developmental norms for the sequencing of language instruction, this language model is based on a logical sequence of programming for practical, functional communication skills (Carrier, 1974).

Symbolic representations—such as pictorial symbols, photographs, and verbal symbols (the alphabet)—have been used with severely retarded children and physically handicapped individuals. Generally, these representations are arranged on a communication board (McDonald, 1975a) and placed on display in front of the individual. To achieve a communicative act, such as expressing hunger, the individual simply points (or gestures in some way) to the representation on the communication board (see Figure 6–1).

Two language systems in general use for communication boards are Rebus and Blissymbolics. Rebus is a nonspeech communication system based on symbols that represent entire words or parts of words (C.R. Clark, Davies, & Woodcock, 1974). Rebus forms are either pictographic (concrete picture representations) or geometric (abstract) (see Figure 6–2). Rebus symbols have recently been used to facilitate international communication. Road signs are an example of such international usage. Rebus has also been used to teach young children to read and has been adapted for use with the nonverbal child.

Blissymbolics was developed in 1942 by Charles K. Bliss. It was meant to be an international written language to help overcome world communication problems (Archer, 1977). Although it was not originally intended for use with the handicapped, it has gained wide usage for that purpose since 1971, when it was adapted for nonverbal children (McNaughton, 1975).

Blissymbolics is a graphic symbol system that employs the development of logical forms to communicate meaning (see Figure 6–3). A relatively small number of symbol elements are combined in a logical system to represent thousands of meanings (McDonald, 1980). The advantage of this

Figure 6–1 A Communication Board

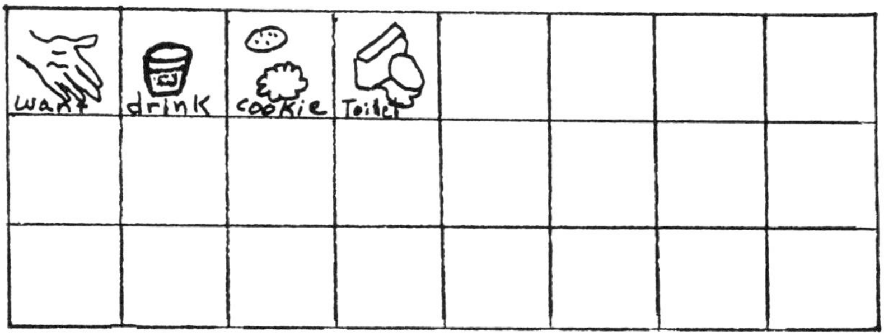

Figure 6–2 Rebus Symbols

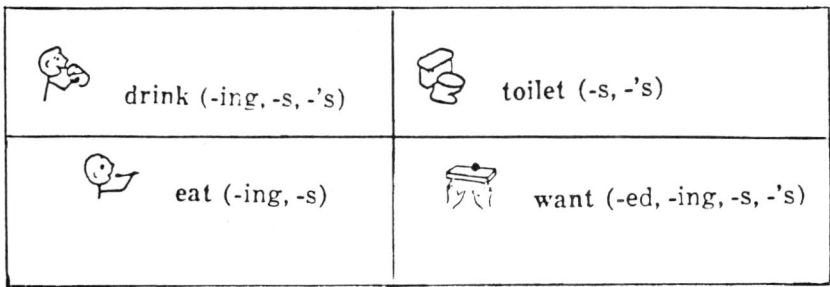

Figure 6–3 Blissymbols

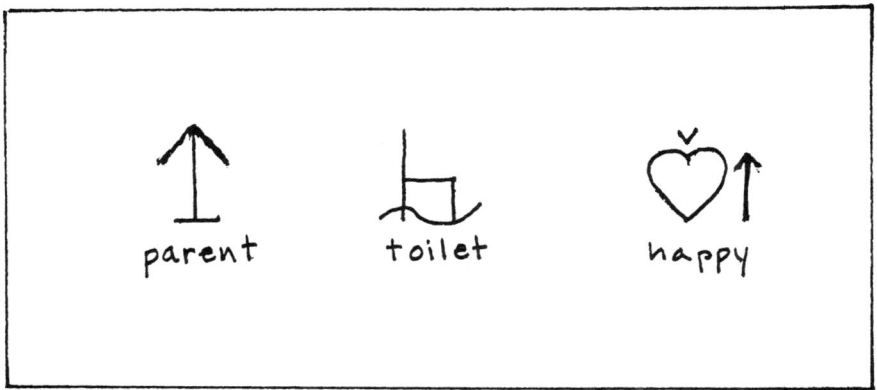

representational system over other systems is that an infinite number of original communicative utterances can be expressed by combining the symbolic units. It is maximally useful for those handicapped individuals who are capable of learning an elaborate grammatical language system.

Traditional orthography is a system of communication that involves the written word. Its effectiveness with autistic children was demonstrated by LaVigna (1977). As a form of representation, traditional orthography offers an advantage over other systems in that it is more readily understood by the general population. It is a system used and recognized by most adults with whom the child will come into contact. Use of the system, however, requires cognitive abilities beyond those of most nonverbal autistic children. The number of autistic children who might benefit from traditional orthography is therefore limited.

Nonoral communication systems, whether they are manual signs or other symbol systems, require individual assessment to determine which, if any, are appropriate for the autistic child. Prerequisite skills are necessary. The child must be able to pay attention to visual stimuli; also the child must be able to point, signal, or use manual gestures. Above all, the child must desire to communicate. Instruction in attending should precede any attempts to teach communication. When the child achieves success in communicating and receives positive reinforcement in the form of responses from the environment, motivation to communicate is enhanced.

The Use of Manual Signs To Teach Communication

Relevant Studies

In recent years, an increasing number of studies have demonstrated the effectiveness of teaching communication to autistic children through manual signing. Though most of these studies are case reports and deal with a limited number of subjects, they have shown that severely dysfunctional, nonverbal autistic children can be taught to communicate (Bonvillian & Nelson, 1976; Carr, Binkoff, Kologinsky, & Eddy, 1978; Creedon, 1973; Dores & Carr, 1979; Konstantareas, Hunter, & Sloman, 1982; Salvin, Routh, Foster, & Lovejoy, 1977; Stull, Edkins, Krause, McGavin, Brand, & Webster, 1980; Webster, McPherson, Sloman, Evans, & Fruchter, 1973). Manual signs have proved to be an effective communication training tool where other modes of communication have failed (Salvin et al., 1977). Manual gestures and signs have been used alone (Barrera, Lobato-Barrera, & Sulzer-Azaroff, 1980; Daniloff & Shafer, 1981) and in combination with spoken words (Barrera et al., 1980; Benaroya, Wesley, Ogilvie, Klein, & Meany, 1977; M. Cohen, 1979; Konstantareas, Webster, & Oxman, 1980; Krug, Arick, Scanlon, Almond, Rosenblum, & Border, 1979). In some cases, while the initial communication training involved the use of manual signs, the children transferred their newly acquired skill into verbal communication (Benaroya et al., 1977; M. Cohen, 1979; Fulwiler & Fouts, 1976; A.M. Miller & E.E. Miller, 1973). These children seemed to use manual communication as a vehicle for speech.

Manual communication has also been used to teach verbal autistic children to overcome difficult discriminations between polar concepts, such as yes and no (Hinerman, Walker, & Jenson, 1979). Sign language has also been used with echolalic children to increase relevant spontaneous speech (M. Cohen, 1979). Most studies report the efficacy of using manual communication techniques with mute or nonverbal autistic children. For most of these children, manual communication represents a first attempt at any type of interaction. The studies have not, as yet, reported the acquisition of an expanded linguistic system; that is, the subjects did not acquire age-appropriate language usage as a result of manual communication. However, some children did acquire an expanded vocabulary of signed words that were ultimately used spontaneously. Since communication, rather than language usage comparable to adult grammar, is critical for the autistic child, manual communication seems to be appropriate and desirable in many cases.

The social and behavioral advantages offered by manual communication were demonstrated by Casey (1978) and Fulwiler and Fouts (1976). In these studies, autistic children who learned to communicate for the first time through manual signs showed increased social interaction and decreased inappropriate behaviors that generalized to the total environment.

Types of Systems

Various types of manual communication systems have been used to teach language to autistic children. American sign language (ASL) or a modified version of ASL is probably the most widely used system, though not necessarily the most appropriate. ASL has been in existence since 1817 (Moores, 1980). It was developed to assist the deaf and the hearing impaired in the use of language to communicate with others (Watson, 1973). ASL is used by the majority of deaf adults in the United States (Moores, 1981).

Since ASL has its roots in French sign language and the Spanish manual alphabet (Moores, 1980), the gestural symbol system sometimes deviates from the grammatical structure of English. ASL is composed of manually produced visual symbols (signs) that stand for words or concepts used in spoken language (Thorpe, 1972) (see Figure 6–4). However, the arrangement of signs in a sentence may occur in the same order as in English or they may occur in a different order. Generally, when ASL is used with the autistic population, it is modified to be coordinated with speech, and the word order follows that of English (Moores, 1981).

American sign language is a language system in itself; therefore, any modification must permit the simultaneous transmission of signed and spoken words. This relegates the system to a substitution of signs as a

Figure 6–4 American Sign Language (ASL)

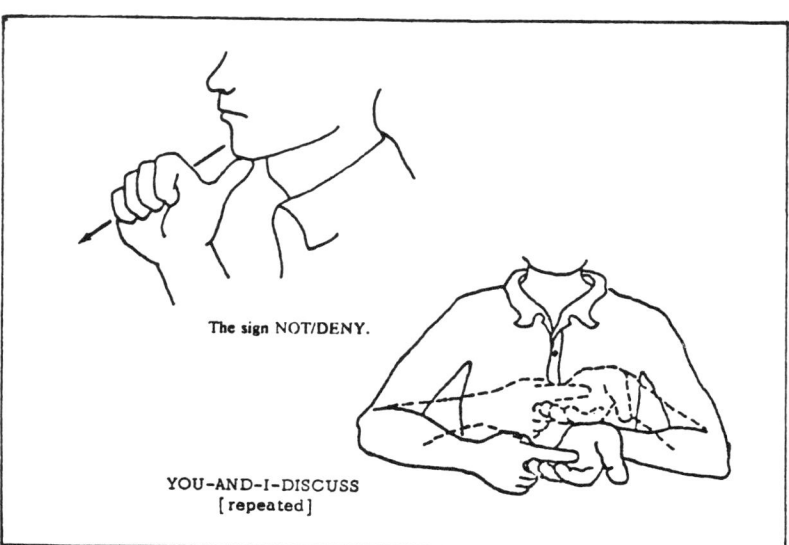

The sign NOT/DENY.

YOU–AND–I–DISCUSS
[repeated]

Source: Reprinted from *American Sign Language and Sign Systems* by R.B. Wilbur, with permission of University Park Press, Baltimore, Md., © 1979; and from *Lexical Borrowing in American Sign Language* by R. Battison, with permission of the author, © 1978 by Linstock Press, Silver Spring, Md.

code for words being spoken (Stokoe, 1980). Since autistic subjects, so far, use fewer words and their signed utterances are less complex than when used by the deaf, such a modification of ASL seems appropriate. However, since ASL is not a one-to-one substitution for the spoken word, its use is more appropriate for children who have the potential to develop a communication system that approaches spoken English in flexibility, efficiency, and complexity. The candidate for ASL must possess the cognitive capacity to learn a language system (Silverman, 1980). Unless modifications are made, ASL is not appropriate for nonverbal autistic children.

An alternative to ASL is signing exact English (SEE) (Gustason, Pfetzing, & Zawolkow, 1980). SEE was developed in 1969 for use with the young deaf child. It was created in an effort to overcome the educational retardation of deaf students. SEE represents an attempt to make signing compatible with English by providing a more direct translation of spoken English into visual symbols. In contrast to American sign language, which is idea-based, signing exact English is a word-based system (Hollis & Carrier, 1978) (see Figure 6–5).

Figure 6–5 Signing Exact English

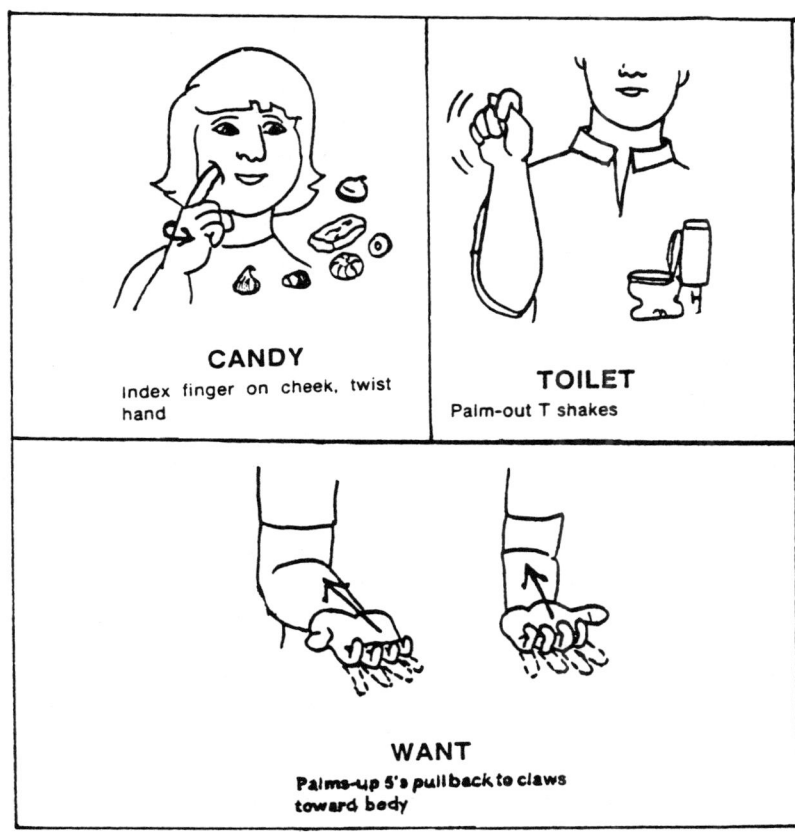

CANDY
Index finger on cheek, twist hand

TOILET
Palm-out T shakes

WANT
Palms-up 5's pull back to claws toward body

Source: Reprinted from *Signing Exact English* by G. Gustason, D. Pfetzing, and E. Zawolkow, with permission of Modern Signs Press, Los Alamitos, Calif., © 1980.

SEE is not widely used by the deaf community. However, there are advantages in using this system with the very young child, particularly the mentally retarded or developmentally delayed child. The shape and configuration of the signs in SEE bear a concrete resemblance to their corresponding words, wherever possible. This is particularly helpful for autistic children, for whom the visual image, or iconicity, is important for perceptual processing and retention of information (Siple, Hatfield, & Caccamise, 1978). In addition to iconicity, SEE has the potential for word-for-word translation. Since simultaneous communication is the preferred mode with educators of autistic children, SEE would seem to be preferable to other manual communication systems. The rationale for using SEE is that the young child will see and use actual English. For deaf children of normal intelligence, this could mean the development of language that is comparable to that of hearing children (Hollis & Carrier, 1978). For developmentally delayed, retarded, and autistic children, it could mean the acquisition of at least the fundamentals of communication.

Advantages

Traditionally, language training programs for autistic children have focused on the development of oral communication. Procedures such as those used by Lovaas (1977) and Lovaas, Berberich, Perloff, and Schaeffer (1966) are effective with echolalic or minimally verbal children. However, an alternative mode may be necessary for the mute child.

Manual communication is an accepted form of natural communication (Gallaudet, 1980). Manual signs are visible. They are in the natural company of facial expressions, eye and body movements, posture movements, and other gestures. Visual communication is natural in interaction between humans. Thus, the visual system gives mute autistic children a means to communicate and makes them members of the human community.

Visual communication with signs seems to be advantageous for some autistic individuals who have difficulty with processing auditory information. Some autistic children who have difficulty imitating speech can be taught to respond motorically. In some cases, simultaneous communication (pairing signs with spoken words) facilitates speech. Thus, manual communication may be used to substitute, develop, supplement, or strengthen verbal language skills.

The physical characteristics of manual signs allow for easy manipulation. This can be essential in the early stages of learning, since prompting and shaping are often necessary in order to establish responding behavior in autistic children.

Most nonverbal children can learn at least a few signs and therefore can communicate basic needs and desires. By providing the child with a means for expressing needs, the foundation of functional communication is established. Eisenberg (1956) and Rutter (1978b) have noted that functional language is an indicator of prognosis for the autistic child. It has also been demonstrated that the development of communication skills can lead to improvement in adaptive and social skills. If autistic children can be taught to use some form of communication, their behavior problems tend to diminish (L. Wing, 1979).

Although verbal training is successful with some autistic children, it is often frustrating and costly in terms of valuable time spent. The autistic child does not have time to waste. If verbal imitation is not immediately effective (about four to six weeks is enough time to determine whether or not the child will be able to use speech), an alternative mode should be used (Carr, 1980). The fact that many autistic children do learn to use manual signs indicates that they are capable of some type of communication.

Manual communication provides a nonauditory medium for expression, which in turn provides the user with a response from the environment. Reinforcement for communication thus provides motivation for continued social interaction. The use of manual signs may limit the child to communication with a select group of communicating partners; yet the ability to communicate at all may depend upon the mode of communication that is selected.

Appendix 6–B contains detailed instructions for a manual communication program that may be used to teach the nonverbal autistic child to communicate. Activities for each step in the program are presented in Table 6B–1. This program should be used only after the child has learned to imitate motor movements. (An additional program form for teacher use is provided in Appendix C.)

SUMMARY

Language, speech, and communication are terms that have related, but different, meanings. Language is the system of rules used by a group of people to express ideas or concepts. Speech is an outward (vocal) manifestation or expression of language. Communication implies a relationship between individuals in which ideas and concepts are shared. Language, speech, and communication all have complex rules that govern their usage; however, communication may be regarded as the least complex, and most primitive, of the three. It can occur even in the absence of language and speech.

Autistic children are typically noncommunicative; they fail to develop the most primitive rules for sharing in exchanges of information.

Assessing the communicative abilities of autistic children begins with close observation of purposeful attempts to engage others in some reciprocal (shared) event. Observation of the child's responses to the environment leads the instructor to develop goals that will reflect the child's need to communicate. Assessment procedures lead the instructor to determine if the child will be able to learn to use spoken language (speech) or if alternative modes of communication need to be taught. Selection criteria for determining the first words to be taught should be based on the words' functions and usefulness for the child.

Imitation is the first step in teaching autistic children to communicate. The procedure for teaching imitation begins with physically prompting the desired behavior. The amount of physical guidance is then systematically reduced until the child independently matches the adult's model.

Imitation training begins with teaching the child to imitate motor activities. First, imitation of gross motor actions is taught; this is followed by imitation of fine motor actions. Next, imitation of sounds used in speech is taught. Imitation of alternative types of expression (such as manual signs or gestures) is taught when the child fails to imitate speech sounds. Nonspeech communication systems include gestures, sign language, pointing to pictures or symbolic representations, graphic symbols or written words, and writing. The use of manual gestures and sign language has proven effective in teaching some autistic children to communicate.

Appendix 6–A

Instructions and Format for Implementing an Imitation Training Program

INSTRUCTIONS FOR IMITATION

Goal

The child will imitate the model when the instructor says, "Do this."

Setting

The imitation session will be conducted in a variety of settings.

Materials

Two small chairs facing each other, a small table beside the instructor's chair (or the instructor and child may sit on the floor facing each other), a written program, extra data sheets, a pencil, and backup reinforcers.

Criterion for Mastery

Eighty percent correct in 40 trials.

Procedures for the Delivery of Consequences

Reinforcement

Following each correct response, the instructor gives the child social reinforcement and backup reinforcement.

Punishment

Following each incorrect response, the instructor withholds reinforcement. The instructor breaks eye contact with the child and turns away for about five seconds.

Activities

Using the activities listed in Table 6A–1, teach the child to imitate five gross motor actions and ten fine motor actions. List the gross motor actions to be taught:

1. _____
2. _____
3. _____
4. _____
5. _____

List the fine motor actions to be taught:

1. _____
2. _____
3. _____
4. _____
5. _____
6. _____
7. _____
8. _____
9. _____
10. _____

Table 6A–1 Component Activities of an Imitation Program

PROGRAM: MOTOR IMITATION
Step 1

Stimulus	Prompt	Response	Consequence	Data
1. Instructor says, "Do this."				Session 1: Date _____ % Correct _____
2. Instructor demonstrates action.				Session 2: Date _____ % Correct _____
	3. Instructor gives full manual guidance.			Session 3: Date _____ % Correct _____
		4. Child complies with prompt.		
			5. Instructor delivers social and backup reinforcement.	Session 4: Date _____ % Correct _____
		6. Child resists prompt.		
			7. Instructor implements punishment.	

Table 6A–1 continued

PROGRAM: MOTOR IMITATION
Step 2

Stimulus	Prompt	Response	Consequence	Data
1. Instructor says, "Do this."				Session 1: Date _____ % Correct _____
2. Instructor demonstrates action.				
	3. Instructor partially guides child to complete action.			Session 2: Date _____ % Correct _____
		4. Child completes imitative action.		
			5. Instructor delivers social and backup reinforcement.	Session 3: Date _____ % Correct _____
		6. Child does not complete action.		
			7. Instructor implements punishment.	Session 4: Date _____ % Correct _____

PROGRAM: MOTOR IMITATION

Step 3

1. Instructor says, "Do this."

2. Instructor demonstrates action.

3. Child imitates action.

4. Instructor delivers social and backup reinforcement.

5. Child does not imitate action.

6. Instructor implements punishment.

Session 1:
Date _____
% Correct _____

Session 2:
Date _____
% Correct _____

Session 3:
Date _____
% Correct _____

Session 4:
Date _____
% Correct _____

Appendix 6–B

Instructions and Format for Implementing a Manual Communication Program

INSTRUCTIONS FOR MANUAL COMMUNICATION

Goal

When shown a food item or an object, the child will produce the manual sign for the object.

Setting

The communication session will be conducted in a variety of settings.

Materials

Two small chairs facing each other, a small table beside the instructor's chair (or the instructor and child may sit on the floor or stand facing each other), a written program, extra data sheets, a pencil, stimulus items or objects, and additional backup reinforcers.

Criterion for Mastery

Eighty percent correct in 40 trials.

Procedures for the Delivery of Consequences

Reinforcement

Following each correct response, the instructor gives the child social reinforcement and backup reinforcement. Whenever possible, the stimulus item is the backup reinforcer.

Punishment

Following each incorrect response, the instructor withholds reinforcement. The instructor breaks eye contact with the child and turns away for about five seconds.

Activities

Using the activities in Table 6B–1, teach the child to produce the manual sign for the stimulus item. List the vocabulary signs to be taught:

(e.g., candy) _____

_____

_____

_____

_____

_____

Table 6B–1 Component Activities of a Manual Communication Program

PROGRAM: MANUAL COMMUNICATION
Step 1

Stimulus	Prompt	Response	Consequence	Data
1. Instructor shows child (candy).				Session 1: Date _____ % Correct _____
2. Instructor says, "What's this? Say, ('candy')."				Session 2: Date _____ % Correct _____
3. Instructor demonstrates sign for (candy).				Session 3: Date _____ % Correct _____
	4. Instructor gives full manual guidance.	5. Child complies with prompt.	6. Instructor delivers social reinforcement and (candy).	Session 4: Date _____ % Correct _____
		7. Child resists prompt.	8. Instructor implements punishment.	

PROGRAM: MANUAL COMMUNICATION
Step 2

	Session 1: Date _____ % Correct _____	Session 2: Date _____ % Correct _____	Session 3: Date _____ % Correct _____	Session 4: Date _____ % Correct _____
1. Instructor shows child (candy).				
2. Instructor says, "What's this? Say, ('candy')."				
3. Instructor demonstrates sign for (candy).				
4. Instructor partially guides child to produce sign for (candy).				
5. Child produces sign for (candy).				
6. Instructor delivers social reinforcement and (candy).				
7. Child does not produce sign for (candy).				
8. Instructor implements punishment.				

Table 6B–1 continued

PROGRAM: MANUAL COMMUNICATION
Step 3

Stimulus	Prompt	Response	Consequence	Data
1. Instructor shows child (candy).				Session 1: Date___ [grid] % Correct___
2. Instructor says, "What's this? Say, ('candy')."				Session 2: Date___ [grid] % Correct___
3. Instructor demonstrates sign for (candy).				
		4. Child produces sign for (candy).		Session 3: Date___ [grid] % Correct___
			5. Instructor delivers social reinforcement and (candy).	
		6. Child does not produce sign for (candy).		Session 4: Date___ [grid] % Correct___
			7. Instructor implements punishment.	

PROGRAM: MANUAL COMMUNICATION
Step 4

		Session 1: Date _____ ☐☐☐☐ % Correct _____	Session 2: Date _____ ☐☐☐☐ % Correct _____	Session 3: Date _____ ☐☐☐☐ % Correct _____	Session 4: Date _____ ☐☐☐☐ % Correct _____
1. Instructor shows child (candy).					
2. Instructor says, "What's this? Say, ('candy')."					
	3. Child produces sign for (candy).				
		4. Instructor delivers social reinforcement and (candy).			
	5. Child does not produce sign for (candy).				
		6. Instructor implements punishment.			

Table 6B–1 continued

PROGRAM: MANUAL COMMUNICATION
Step 5

Stimulus	Prompt	Response	Consequence	Data
1. Instructor shows child (candy).				Session 1: Date ___ % Correct ___
2. Instructor says, "What's this?"				Session 2: Date ___ % Correct ___
		3. Child produces sign for (candy).	4. Instructor delivers social reinforcement and (candy).	Session 3: Date ___ % Correct ___
		5. Child does not produce sign for (candy).	6. Instructor implements punishment.	Session 4: Date ___ % Correct ___

PROGRAM: MANUAL COMMUNICATION
Step 6

			Session 1: Date _____ % Correct _____	Session 2: Date _____ % Correct _____	Session 3: Date _____ % Correct _____	Session 4: Date _____ % Correct _____
1. Instructor shows child (candy).						
	2. Child produces sign for (candy).					
		3. Instructor delivers social reinforcement and (candy).				
	4. Child does not produce sign for (candy).					
		5. Instructor implements punishment.				

Table 6B–1 continued

PROGRAM: MANUAL COMMUNICATION
Step 7

Stimulus	Prompt	Response	Consequence	Data
1. Instructor places (candy) and one other item in front of child. Instructor points to (candy).				Session 1: Date_____ % Correct_____
		2. Child produces sign for (candy).		Session 2: Date_____ % Correct_____
			3. Instructor delivers social reinforcement and (candy).	Session 3: Date_____ % Correct_____
		4. Child does not produce sign for (candy).		Session 4: Date_____ % Correct_____
			5. Instructor implements punishment.	

PROGRAM: MANUAL COMMUNICATION
Step 8

			Session 1: Date _____ [grid] % Correct _____	Session 2: Date _____ [grid] % Correct _____	Session 3: Date _____ [grid] % Correct _____	Session 4: Date _____ [grid] % Correct _____
1. Instructor shows child (candy), then hides it.	2. Child produces sign for (candy).	3. Instructor delivers social reinforcement and (candy).				
	4. Child does not produce sign for (candy).	5. Instructor implements punishment.				

Chapter 7

Using Overcorrection
To Teach Manual
Communication

Many autistic children never learn to speak; many never learn to use language. Most, however, can learn to communicate. Lovaas (1968) has demonstrated that autistic children who can learn to imitate sounds can learn to use speech to communicate. (Programs for teaching children to imitate were presented in Chapter 6.) When a child fails to achieve the level of proficiency necessary to complete imitation programs, the methods of instruction must be modified. In spite of the child's capacity to produce sounds, attempts to teach the child to produce sequenced speech sounds and to formulate words may fail. Often, nonverbal, noncommunicative autistic children simply do not imitate. Prompting and prompt fading, shaping, and modeling do not seem to work. Attempts to teach motor imitation fail, as do attempts to teach verbal imitation. In such cases, a procedure such as overcorrection can be useful.

This chapter presents a program that combines manual communication with positive practice overcorrection to teach the profoundly noncommunicating child a few responses that can, in some cases, be expanded to give the child a number of expressive signs. Manual communication is used in this program for a number of reasons. Manual signs are visible; they can be seen by the child. Unlike auditory messages, signs are spatial; they give the child the advantage of being able to observe the stimulus for a longer period of time. The concrete nature of manual signs allows the instructor to manipulate or to prompt physically the correct response.

IMPLEMENTING THE PROGRAM

The signs used in the program we present here are signing exact English (SEE) (Gustason et al., 1980). SEE is used because of the iconicity of its signs; that is, the configuration of each sign resembles a quality or association attached to the word it represents. For example, the sign for milk is made with a closed fist held vertically. The fist opens and closes slightly to simulate the action of milking a cow (see Figure 7–1).

Overcorrection is used because of its value as a procedure to reduce inappropriate responses while teaching the correct response. Requiring the child to practice the correct response each time a failure occurs has obvious instructional value. The extended practice and manual guidance involved in the overcorrection procedure requires additional effort by the child. Presumably, the child learns that it is easier to produce the correct response than to carry out the extended practice.

An Illustrative Study

The effectiveness of the above procedure was demonstrated with an eight-year-old autistic boy (Hinerman, Jenson, Walker, & Petersen, 1982). Previous efforts to teach the child to imitate motor responses through prompting and modeling had failed, as had attempts to teach the child to use speech. The child did not use any form of communication. The goal of the program was to teach the child to use a few manual signs to express his needs and desires. The very structured procedures were used until the child was proficient in producing the signs on command. Then, less stringent means were used to test for generalization and spontaneous usage.

Tasks and Procedures

The study consisted of teaching the subject to label two objects using the correct manual sign. Each task was taught separately in discrete trials. In Task A, the subject was required to match the manual sign for milk to a glass of milk. In Task B, the subject was required to match the manual sign for cookie to a cookie (see Figures 7–1 and 7–2 for the SEE signs for milk and cookie).

The baseline was established in three sessions of 20 trials each. In each trial the subject was shown a glass of milk (Task A) or a cookie (Task B). The experimenter said, "What's this? Say, 'milk' " (for Task A), or, "What's this? Say, 'cookie' " (for Task B). The experimenter then gave the manual sign for milk (Task A) or cookie (Task B). A response was scored a plus (+) when the subject correctly imitated the manual sign, and the subject was rewarded with social reinforcement (praise), a drink of milk, and a piece of cookie. Each incorrect response was scored a minus (−) and was ignored.

Intervention was implemented at three levels of mastery. Trials for Level I were the same as those for the baseline, except that, when the

Figure 7–1 Sign for Milk in Signing Exact English (SEE)

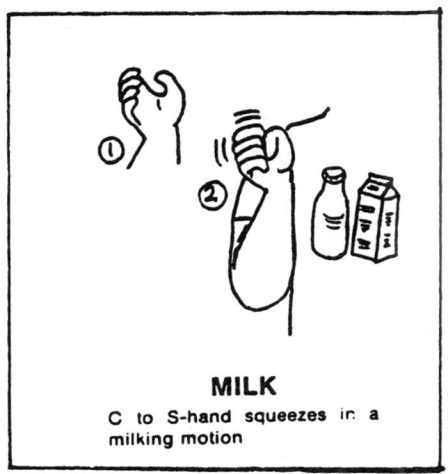

MILK

C to S-hand squeezes in a
milking motion

Source: Reprinted from *Signing Exact English* by G. Gustason, D. Pfetzing, and E. Zawolkow, with permission of Modern Signs Press, Los Alamitos, Calif., © 1980.

Figure 7–2 Sign for Cookie in Signing Exact English (SEE)

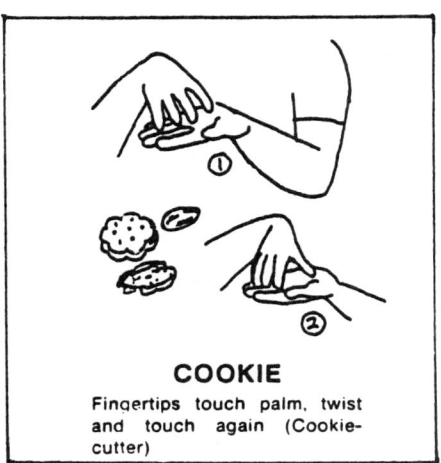

COOKIE

Fingertips touch palm, twist
and touch again (Cookie-
cutter)

Source: Reprinted from *Signing Exact English* by G. Gustason, D. Pfetzing, and E. Zawolkow, with permission of Modern Signs Press, Los Alamitos, Calif., © 1980.

subject gave an incorrect response, he was physically guided to form the manual sign ten times (positive practice overcorrection). Tables 7–1 and 7–2 illustrate the procedures used to teach the manual signs and the number of trials it took to reach the criterion. As the subject assumed more responsibility in making the sign, the experimenter's physical guidance was gradually reduced. Correct responses were rewarded with social praise and the edible reinforcer (a drink of milk and a piece of cookie).

In Level II, the subject was shown a glass of milk (Task A) or a cookie (Task B). The experimenter said, "What's this? Say, 'milk,' " or, "What's this? Say, 'cookie.' " The imitative model (the manual sign) was omitted in Level II. The subject was required to produce the correct manual sign following the stimulus. Correct responses were rewarded with social praise and the edible reinforcer. Incorrect responses were followed by positive practice overcorrection (as in Level I).

In Level III, the subject was shown a glass of milk or a cookie. The experimenter said, "What's this?" The verbal prompt ("say, 'milk,' " or "say, 'cookie' ") was omitted in Level III. The subject was required to give the manual sign for milk or cookie, depending on the task. Consequences for correct and incorrect responses were the same as for Levels I and II.

When the subject had mastered the labeling task for both milk and cookie, the items were presented randomly. The experimenter said, "What's this?" and the subject was required to produce the correct sign. The consequences were the same as those in previous tasks. The procedures for teaching the child to respond to random presentation and the number of trials it took to reach mastery are shown in Table 7–3.

Delivery of the primary reinforcer (milk and cookie) was thinned as the subject achieved the predetermined level of mastery. The criterion for moving from one level to the next and for thinning of the reinforcement schedule was 80 percent or better for 60 trials.

Results

In the study, the subject's correct response rate at baseline was zero percent. When the subject was asked, "What's this?" given the verbal prompt, "Say, 'milk' " or "Say, 'cookie,' " and was shown the model for the corresponding manual sign, the subject failed to imitate the sign.

When the intervention (positive practice overcorrection) was implemented for Task A (milk), it took the subject 400 trials across 20 days to reach Level I, it took 140 trials across 7 days to reach Level II, and it took 200 trials across 11 days to reach Level III. When the intervention was implemented for Task B (cookie), it took the subject 960 trials across 48

Table 7–1 Procedures for Using Overcorrection To Teach the Manual Sign for Milk and To Label the Item

TASK A: MILK

Baseline:

Stimulus	Response	Consequence	Criterion for Mastery	# Trials to Criterion
Visual: Glass of milk Verbal: "What's this? Say 'milk'" Visual: Manual sign for milk	Manual sign for milk	Correct response: social reinforcement, milk and cookie Incorrect response: ignore	60 trials at 0%	60

Intervention: Level I

Stimulus	Response	Consequence	Criterion for Mastery	# Trials to Criterion
Visual: Glass of milk Verbal: "What's this? Say 'milk'" Visual: Manual sign for milk	Manual sign for milk	Correct response. social reinforcement, milk and cookie Incorrect response: ten positive practices (overcorrection)	80% correct for 60 trials	400

Table 7-1 continued

Intervention: Level II

Stimulus	Response	Consequence	Criterion for Mastery	#Trials to Criterion
Visual: Glass of milk Verbal: "What's this? Say, 'milk' " (no model)	Manual sign for milk	Correct response: social reinforcement, milk and cookie Incorrect response: ten positive practices	80% correct for 60 trials	140

Intervention: Level III

Stimulus	Response	Consequence	Criterion for Mastery	# Trials to Criterion
Visual: Glass of milk Verbal: "What's this?" (no model)	Manual sign for milk	Correct response: social reinforcement, milk and cookie Incorrect response: ten positive practices	80% correct for 60 trials	220

Source: Reprinted from "Positive Practice Overcorrection Combined with Additional Procedures To Teach Signed Words to an Autistic Child," by P.S. Hinerman, W.R. Jenson, G.R. Walker, and P.B. Petersen, in the Journal of Autism and Developmental Disorders 12 (1982), with permission of the Plenum Publishing Co., New York.

Table 7–2 Procedures for Using Overcorrection To Teach the Manual Sign for Cookie and To Label the Item

TASK B: COOKIE

Baseline:

Stimulus	Response	Consequence	Criterion for Mastery	# Trials to Criterion
Visual: Cookie Verbal: "What's this? Say 'cookie'" Visual: Manual sign for cookie	Manual sign for cookie	Correct response: social reinforcement, cookie and milk Incorrect response: ignore	60 trials at 0%	60

Intervention: Level I

Stimulus	Response	Consequence	Criterion for Mastery	# Trials to Criterion
Visual: Cookie Verbal: "What's this? Say 'cookie'" Visual: Manual sign for cookie	Manual sign for cookie	Correct response: social reinforcement, cookie and milk Incorrect response: ten positive practices (overcorrection)	80% correct for 60 trials	960

Table 7–2 continued

Intervention: Level II

Stimulus	Response	Consequence	Criterion for Mastery	#Trials to Criterion
Visual: Cookie Verbal: "What's this? Say, 'cookie'" (no model)	Manual sign for cookie	Correct response: social reinforcement, cookie and milk Incorrect response: ten positive practices	80% correct for 60 trials	140

Intervention: Level III

Stimulus	Response	Consequence	Criterion for Mastery	# Trials to Criterion
Visual: Cookie Verbal: "What's this?" (no model)	Manual sign for cookie	Correct response: social reinforcement, cookie and milk Incorrect response: ten positive practices	80% correct for 60 trials	120

Source: Reprinted from "Positive Practice Overcorrection Combined with Additional Procedures To Teach Signed Words to an Autistic Child," by P.S. Hinerman, W.R. Jenson, G.R. Walker, and P.B. Petersen, in the Journal of Autism and Developmental Disorders 12 (1982), with permission of the Plenum Publishing Co., New York.

Table 7-3 Procedures for Using Overcorrection To Teach the Manual Sign for Milk and Cookie in Random Presentations

TASK: RANDOM PRESENTATION OF MILK AND COOKIE

Intervention:

Stimulus	Response	Consequence	Criterion for Mastery	# Trials to Criterion
Visual: Cookie or milk, randomly presented Verbal: "What's this?"	Manual sign for cookie or milk	Correct response: social reinforcement, cookie and milk Incorrect response: ten positive practices	80% correct for 60 trials	220

Source: Reprinted from "Positive Practice Overcorrection Combined with Additional Procedures To Teach Signed Words to an Autistic Child," by P.S. Hinerman, W.R. Jenson, G.R. Walker, and P.B. Petersen, in the *Journal of Autism and Developmental Disorders* 12 (1982), with permission of the Plenum Publishing Co., New York.

days to reach Level I. After 620 trials, the subject was required to practice an unrelated, repetitive task (stand up and sit down), as well as do positive practice. As soon as he reached the criterion, the unrelated task was dropped. It took 140 trials across 7 days to reach Level II; it took 120 trials across 6 days to reach Level III.

When the intervention was implemented for the items presented randomly, it took the subject 220 trials across five days to reach the criterion. Figure 7–3 shows graphically the number of trials required to reach mastery on each level of each task.

As the baseline data indicate, the subject failed to produce or imitate the manual sign for either item. When positive practice overcorrection was implemented, positive results were obtained. When the visual cue (the model for the manual sign) and the verbal instruction (''say, 'milk' '' or, ''say, 'cookie' '') were faded, the subject continued to give the correct sign. Correct labeling on a discrimination task was demonstrated when both stimulus items were randomly presented to the subject.

Conclusions

Manual communication has been shown to be a facilitator in teaching language to autistic children. Some studies have concerned themselves with teaching semimute autistic children to use language effectively, while others have shown that imitative modeling can be used with mute autistic children to teach a simple manual vocabulary. Many mute autistic children, however, are unable to imitate either verbal or visual models. Even when contingent reinforcement is used, these children do not seem to possess the cognitive associations necessary for imitation.

In the study we have presented, the subject had repeatedly failed on verbal and motor imitation tasks, even though past experience indicated that he was highly conditionable on other behavior-shaping tasks. The subject had also been unsuccessful at numerous labeling tasks, which is typical of many autistic children. It appears that the overcorrection procedure was the necessary tool for this particular child to learn imitation of two signs and to use those signs to label their objects appropriately.

The reasons for the success of the intervention are not clear. The overcorrection may have functioned as a boring, repetitive task—a punishment that decreased the rate of incorrect responses. One cannot dismiss, however, the probable effects of repeated practice, combined with intense tactile stimulation and numerous trials. The mode of the manual sign provided a fixed visual cue, whereas the spoken word is a temporary auditory signal. Yet the fact remains that the subject had not previously demonstrated an ability to imitate either visual or auditory signals. Perhaps

Figure 7–3 Graphic Representation of Percentage of Correct Responses in Teaching the Manual Signs for Milk and Cookie Using Overcorrection

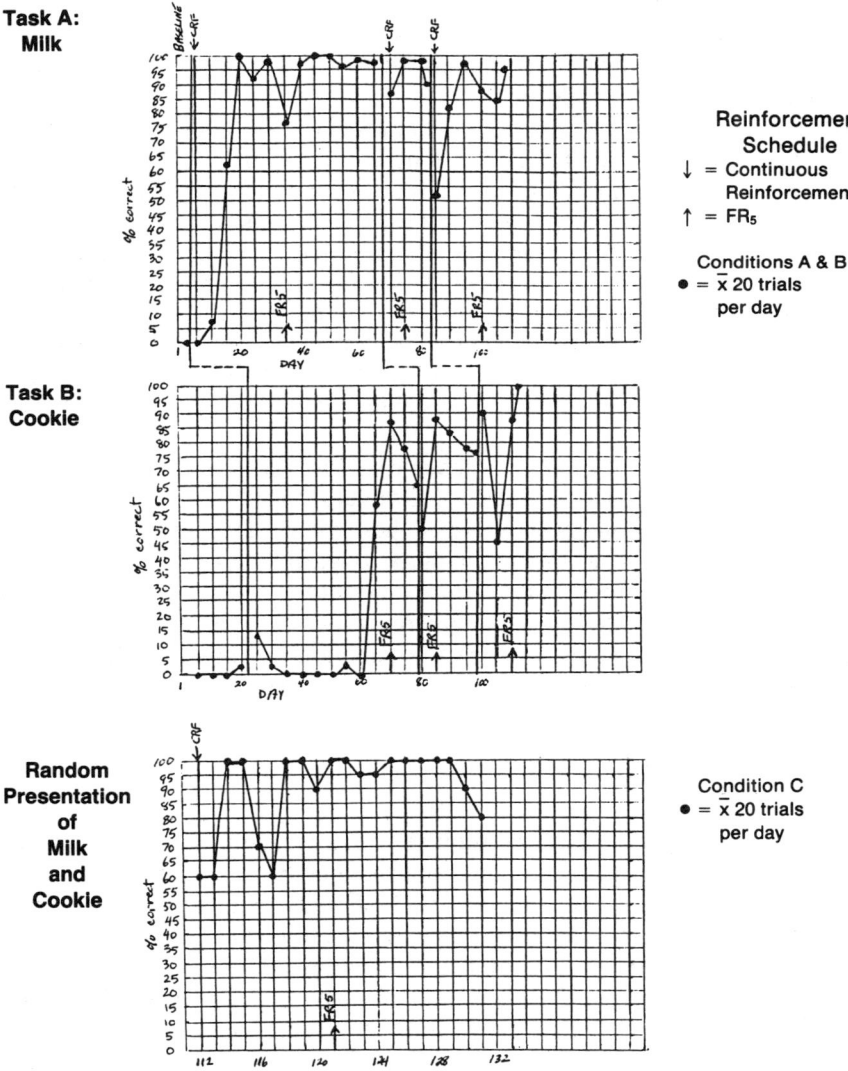

Task A: Milk

Task B: Cookie

Random Presentation of Milk and Cookie

Reinforcement Schedule
↓ = Continuous Reinforcement
↑ = FR₅

Conditions A & B
● = x̄ 20 trials per day

Condition C
● = x̄ 20 trials per day

Source: Reprinted from "Positive Practice Overcorrection Combined with Additional Procedures to Teach Signed Words to an Autistic Child," by P.S. Hinerman, W.R. Jenson, G.R. Walker, and R.B. Peterson, in the *Journal of Autism and Developmental Disorders* 12 (1982), with permission of the Plenum Publishing Co., New York.

the availability of tactile manipulation aided in prompting, whereas verbal and visual cueing are more difficult and less reliable.

The extensive number of trials required to respond correctly to the initial task is typical of the learning rate of autistic children. When the subject finally began to respond correctly, he reached mastery relatively quickly and continued to respond correctly. This learning pattern is not uncommon in autistic children.

One would expect, however, that the second task (cookie) would have been learned more rapidly. There is no evidence that this task was any more difficult; yet the child continued to respond incorrectly for over 900 trials (compared to 400 trials required for the first task). The introduction of the unrelated practice (stand up and sit down), which was intended to punish the incorrect response, coupled with the related practice produced the desired effects. In both tasks, imitation of the sign was acquired slowly and tediously. Once the imitation was established, however, labeling was learned rather quickly. Proof that the child had learned to discriminate was demonstrated when the child was able to label correctly the randomly presented items.

It should not be assumed that these procedures will be effective with all functionally mute autistic children. However, the subject in the study we have presented demonstrates some of the typical learning patterns found in autistic children. Perhaps the inability to learn language through imitation can be initially restructured through overcorrection. The study may also suggest that positive practice overcorrection can be an effective tool for teaching manual signs to some low-functioning autistic children who might otherwise never learn to use functional language.

REQUISITE STEPS

The program presented here requires, as a prerequisite, that the child is able to attend to the instructor. Children who have not been instructed in the attending program (see Chapter 5) should be taught to attend prior to beginning the communication program. Attending behavior is required prior to each discrete trial in the manual communication program.

Directions for "miniattending" by the instructor are presented in Table 7–4. The instructor begins by modeling the correct attending posture. If the child responds by attending (see the definition of attending in chapter 5), the instructor immediately presents the stimulus. If the child does not attend in response to the instructor's model, the instructor verbally directs or manually guides the child to stand up and sit down ten times. This procedure is the same as that of Part IV, Step 5, of the attending program.

Table 7–4 Procedures for Eliciting the Attending Response Prior to Presentation of the Stimulus

TASK: "MINIATTENDING"

Stimulus	Response	Consequence
1. Instructor models attending by sitting with feet on floor, hands on knees, and looking at child.		
	2. Child puts both feet on floor with hands down, is quiet, and looks at instructor for three seconds.	
		3. Instructor presents stimulus.
	4. Child does not keep feet on floor with hands still, is not quiet, or does not look for three seconds.	
		5. Instructor implements overcorrection.

When attending has been achieved, the instructor may use the procedures described in this chapter to instruct the child to use manual signs to label objects. The signs for milk and cookie used in the above program are, of course, for illustrative purposes only. In planning individual programs, the instructor will choose stimulus items that are known to be reinforcing to the child. If the child has not demonstrated a desire for particular objects or activities, it is best to begin with food or liquid items. The instructor may also wish to teach the child the classification rather than the specific names for the items. For example, the sign for food or drink could be taught, and the correct production of the sign could be reinforced by the use of a variety of food or drink items.

Once the child has learned to label correctly a few items that can provide immediate positive reinforcement, the instructor should gradually expand the child's manual vocabulary to include other words that will help the child function in the current and future environment. The instructor should include other edible reinforcers, such as candy, that will be rewarding for the child. Other signs that serve a functional capacity for the child include those for toilet, toy, mother, give, eat (or food), drink, go, and jump. The same discrete trial procedure can be used; and, as new signs are learned, they can be maintained by presenting the items once or twice, interspersed with the new signs. Occasionally, the instructor should present all mastered signs in random order to maintain the child's ability to produce those signs.

As soon as a manual sign is learned, the child should be required to produce that sign at all other appropriate times during the day. For generalization and for spontaneous usage of the manual signs, the instructor should create situations in which the child can use the sign. As more signs are learned, numerous opportunities to use the sign language should be included as a part of the child's daily schedule.

Instructions and a format for implementing a manual communication program using overcorrection are presented in Appendix 7-A. Table 7A-1 lists the requisite activities for each step in the program. An additional blank program form is included in Appendix C. Instructors may wish to use this form to expand a child's manual vocabulary.

SUMMARY

In cases where attempts to teach autistic children to imitate have failed, a combination of manual communication and positive practice overcorrection may provide a means for teaching a few communicative responses. Manual signs are used because they possess visual and tactual properties. They are spatial, they can be seen for as long as necessary, and they can be manipulated by the instructor. Overcorrection is used because of its value in reducing inappropriate responses while teaching the correct response through repetition.

Appendix 7–A

Instructions and Format for Implementing a Manual Communication Program Using Overcorrection

INSTRUCTIONS FOR MANUAL COMMUNICATION USING OVERCORRECTION

Goal

- Part I—The child will produce the manual sign for milk when shown a glass of milk.
- Part II—The child will produce the manual sign for cookie when shown a cookie.
- Part III—The child will produce the manual sign for milk or cookie when the items are presented in random order.

Setting

The sessions will take place in the classroom and other areas of the school. Two small chairs should be placed facing each other. A small table should be placed next to the instructor's chair. All materials should be placed on the table. Edible reinforcers should be placed out of reach of the child. The sessions will be conducted from _____until _____ (filled in by the instructor) daily.

Materials

Two small chairs, a small table, the written program, extra data sheets, a pencil, a glass of milk, a cookie.

Criterion for Mastery

Eighty percent correct in 40 trials.

Procedures for the Delivery of Consequences

Reinforcement

Following each correct response, the instructor gives the child social reinforcement, such as, "Good! You did it!" and a sip of milk or a piece of cookie. The edible reinforcer should be the same as the manual sign produced by the child; for example, if the task is to sign milk, the reinforcer for the correct response should be milk.

Punishment

Following each incorrect response, the instructor implements overcorrection as follows:

- In a firm voice, say, "No, say 'milk' (or 'cookie')."
- Grasp the child's hand(s) and form the correct manual sign.
- Repeat the exercise ten times in succession.
- As the child begins to form the sign, gradually decrease the amount of physical pressure or guidance. Continue to direct the child verbally to practice the sign.
- If the child stops the action or slows down, resume the manual guidance.

Activities

Activities for each part (I–III) and its component steps in the manual communication program, using the manual signs for milk and cookie illustrated in Figures 7–1 and 7–2, are shown in Table 7A–1.

Table 7A–1 Component Activities of a Manual Communication Program Using Overcorrection

PART I: SIGNING FOR MILK
Step 1

Stimulus	Response	Consequence	Data
1. Instructor shows child a glass of milk.			Session 1: Date —— % Correct ——
2. Instructor says, "What's this? Say, 'milk.' "			Session 2: Date —— % Correct ——
3. Instructor demonstrates manual sign for milk.	4. Child imitates manual sign for milk.	5. Instructor gives child social reinforcement and a sip of milk.	Session 3: Date —— % Correct ——
	6. Child does not imitate manual sign for milk.	7. Instructor implements overcorrection.	Session 4: Date —— % Correct ——

Table 7A–1 continued

PART I: SIGNING FOR MILK
Step 2

Stimulus	Response	Consequence	Data
1. Instructor shows child a glass of milk.			Session 1: Date _____ % Correct _____
2. Instructor says, "What's this? Say, 'milk.'"			Session 2: Date _____ % Correct _____
	3. Child produces manual sign for milk.	4. Instructor gives child social reinforcement and a sip of milk.	Session 3: Date _____ % Correct _____
	5. Child does not produce manual sign for milk.	6. Instructor implements overcorrection.	Session 4: Date _____ % Correct _____

PART I: SIGNING FOR MILK
Step 3

		Session 1: Date ———	% Correct ———	Session 2: Date ———	% Correct ———	Session 3: Date ———	% Correct ———	Session 4: Date ———	% Correct ———
1. Instructor shows child a glass of milk.									
2. Instructor says, "What's this?"									
3. Child produces manual sign for milk.									
4. Instructor gives social reinforcement and a sip of milk.									
5. Child does not produce the manual sign for milk.									
6. Instructor implements overcorrection.									

Table 7A–1 continued

PART I: SIGNING FOR MILK
Step 4

Stimulus	Response	Consequence	Data
1. Instructor shows child a glass of milk.			Session 1: Date _____ % Correct _____
	2. Child produces manual sign for milk.		Session 2: Date _____ % Correct _____
		3. Instructor gives child social reinforcement and a sip of milk.	Session 3: Date _____ % Correct _____
	4. Child does not produce manual sign for milk.		Session 4: Date _____ % Correct _____
		5. Instructor implements overcorrection.	

PART II: SIGNING FOR COOKIE
Step 1

		Session 1: Date _____ % Correct _____	Session 2: Date _____ % Correct _____	Session 3: Date _____ % Correct _____	Session 4: Date _____ % Correct _____
1. Instructor places a glass of milk on table, shows child a cookie.					
2. Instructor says, "What's this? Say, 'cookie.'"					
3. Instructor demonstrates manual sign for cookie.					
	4. Child imitates manual sign for cookie.				
5. Instructor gives child social reinforcement and a bite of cookie.					
	6. Child does not imitate manual sign for cookie.				
7. Instructor implements overcorrection.					

Table 7A–1 continued

PART II: SIGNING FOR COOKIE
Step 2

Stimulus	Response	Consequence	Data
1. Instructor places a glass of milk on table, shows child a cookie.			Session 1: Date_____ % Correct_____
2. Instructor says, "What's this? Say, 'cookie.'"			Session 2: Date_____ % Correct_____
	3. Child produces manual sign for cookie.		Session 3: Date_____ % Correct_____
		4. Instructor gives child social reinforcement and a bite of cookie.	Session 4: Date_____ % Correct_____
	5. Child does not produce manual sign for cookie.	6. Instructor implements overcorrection.	

PART II: SIGNING FOR COOKIE
Step 3

		Session 1: Date _____ % Correct _____	Session 2: Date _____ % Correct _____	Session 3: Date _____ % Correct _____	Session 4: Date _____ % Correct _____
1. Instructor places a glass of milk on table, shows child a cookie.					
2. Instructor says, "What's this?"					
3. Child produces manual sign for cookie.	4. Instructor gives child social reinforcement and a bite of cookie.				
5. Child does not produce manual sign for cookie.	6. Instructor implements overcorrection.				

Table 7A–1 continued

PART II: SIGNING FOR COOKIE
Step 4

Stimulus	Response	Consequence	Data
1. Instructor places a glass of milk on table, shows child a cookie.			Session 1: Date _____ % Correct _____
	2. Child produces manual sign for cookie.		Session 2: Date _____ % Correct _____
		3. Instructor gives child social reinforcement and a bite of cookie.	Session 3: Date _____ % Correct _____
	4. Child does not produce manual sign for cookie.		Session 4: Date _____ % Correct _____
		5. Instructor implements overcorrection.	

PART III: SIGNING FOR MILK AND COOKIE
Step 1

			Session 1: Date _____ % Correct _____
1. Instructor shows child milk or cookie, presented in random order.			
	2. Child produces manual sign for milk or cookie.		Session 2: Date _____ % Correct _____
		3. Instructor gives child social reinforcement and edible.	Session 3: Date _____ % Correct _____
	4. Child does not produce correct manual sign.		
		5. Instructor implements overcorrection.	Session 4: Date _____ % Correct _____

Chapter 8

Parental Involvement

Family involvement is an integral part of the autistic child's educational process. Autistic children's needs are not limited to the hours between 9:00 A.M. and 3:00 P.M.; nor are they limited to Monday through Friday, September to June. If autistic children are to be diverted from institutions, an all-out, 24-hour, nonstop effort on the part of parents and professionals is required. To ensure that autistic children reach their full potential as members of the human community, every significant member of the child's environment must be involved in the process. The teaching process must extend beyond the classroom or clinic to include every waking hour of the child's life.

THE CHANGING ROLE OF PARENTS

For years, parents were excluded from participation in therapy. At most, their involvement was confined to psychoanalysis or counseling for themselves. They were left to their own means to find ways of coping with the unmanageable problem behaviors that their autistic children exhibited at home.

Today, parents' roles are changing. Parents are no longer viewed as patients or clients. The new role of the parent is partly the result of studies that have demonstrated that parental attitudes or dispositions do not cause autism (M.K. DeMyer, 1971; Lennox, Callias, & Rutter, 1977; Schopler & Reichler, 1971). The concept of training parents as paraprofessionals to educate, instruct, and treat their autistic children at home is becoming more and more acceptable (Freeman & Ritvo, 1976).

The changing role of parents should not present a threat to professionals. Public Law 94–142 placed education for the handicapped squarely on the shoulders of the public schools. The law also gave parents the right, responsibility, and means to participate in the placement of and development of goals for their children.

The individual education plan (IEP) is the instrument for designating placement and outlining goals. It should reflect a team effort, involving the parents and every professional who works with the child. Special education teachers, speech pathologists, psychologists, social workers, physical therapists, occupational therapists, physicians, and parents should determine together the goals for the child and the best means for achieving those goals.

The IEP planning session should be arranged so that each individual who is involved with the child is permitted to express concerns freely and to suggest goals and treatment methods. However, parents are often, understandably, intimidated by hordes of professionals gathered around a very formal-looking table. But professionals who are conscious of the feelings of parents will encourage and support their contributions. Valuable information can be gained during the IEP meeting by encouraging parents to set short-term and long-term goals for their children.

SETTING GOALS

Setting goals is important for several reasons. It is critical to the analysis of progress. Goals help teachers and parents to see where the child is, to remember where the child has been, and to judge how far the child will go. The process of setting long-term goals may be crucial to parental involvement in the child's program. It is often difficult for parents to be consistent in responding to their children's behaviors. The benefits of the day-to-day management of behavior problems can be obscured by the constant effort required just to keep the child from falling farther behind.

It is also a hard task for parents to force their children constantly to learn skills that will be essential if the child is to remain at home or in the community. Young handicapped children evoke sympathy. Many well-meaning adults inadvertently teach handicapped children to be dependent upon the adults. They try to help by doing for the child instead of helping the child learn to act independently. Professionals can provide a service to parents in this regard by guiding them through the goal-setting process. Setting long-term goals can help parents understand why strict procedures are necessary, and how such procedures will ultimately benefit the child.

Consider, for example, the 6-year-old autistic girl who refused to dress herself. The child would throw violent tantrums whenever anyone tried to prompt her to dress herself; yet she would submissively allow her mother to dress her. Of course, it was much easier for the mother to dress this small, cute little girl than to go through the tantrums and fighting to get her to dress herself. It had not occurred to the mother that she was teaching her daughter to be dependent upon her. It had not occurred to her that, at the age of 20, or even 40, this child might still need someone to dress her. The thought of a 6-year-old girl needing help in dressing was not so bad, but the prospect of a 20-year-old woman having to be dressed by another adult was enough to make the mother in this case select "self-help: dressing" as a goal for her child.

From the time the child is first diagnosed, the parents should be encouraged to plan for future placement. If the parents want to keep their autistic child at home, the child will have to become competent in certain skills. Problem behaviors will have to be eliminated, and functional, adaptive skills will have to be taught. The parents, too, will have to learn new skills for working with and managing their child. Professionals can provide a tremendous service to parents by helping them plan realistic goals for their autistic children and by giving them the tools for achieving those goals. Parents cannot be expected to perform the same role as teachers or therapists, but they can be valuable partners in the educational process.

PARENT TRAINING

An active role for parents is an essential element in an effective program for autistic children. When parents are trained to manage behaviors and to supplement teaching efforts by working with the child at home, the chances of an autistic child remaining at home are increased (Freeman & Ritvo, 1976). Lovaas (1978) has demonstrated that children whose parents were trained to carry out behavior therapy continued to improve. This illustrates the value of training parents to be coeducators.

Professionals will always be confronted with the problem of motivating parents who, for one reason or another, avoid involvement. Parents of autistic children experience burnout, just as teachers do. By the time an autistic child is six years old, the parents have gotten the runaround from so many professionals that they feel frustrated or demoralized. They have usually been given several diagnoses, including, "He'll grow out of it," "She's retarded," "He has an emotional problem," or, finally, "There's nothing we can do."

Parents experience anger, frustration, depression, and bitterness at various times in their lives, or all at once. They experience the never-ending agony of knocking on legislative and administrative doors to obtain money for services. Inevitably, they are placed on waiting lists for months—even years. At some point, parents want to rest; they just do not want to be involved.

Yet, while it is still the teacher's responsibility to educate the child, and the success of an educational program cannot depend upon parental involvement, parent participation can enhance the program and can have a considerable effect on the child's rate of progress. Therefore, it is for the benefit of the child that the professionals try to build relationships with the parents.

Parent-Professional Collaboration

Frequent collaboration between the professionals and the parents about target behaviors and goals is a good way to begin. The first objective of a close home-and-school relationship should be to select a behavior that the parents have long desired their child to accomplish, or to select a problem behavior that the parents desperately desire to change. When the parents experience success in teaching the child a new skill, or in eliminating a problem behavior, they will be more likely to continue to participate (Kyne, 1980).

In order for parents to become coeducators, parent training must be incorporated into the child's educational program. Parent training can be extended to include learning behavior management techniques, conducting discrete trial sessions, conducting nondiscrete trial sessions, and developing programs for teaching new skills. Parent training can also be minimal, but still provide the parents with enough information and practice to enable them to implement behavior management techniques in the home.

Parent participation will depend on the parents' time, motivation, and previous experience with professionals. In this context, the professional's responsibility must be to encourage, not coerce. Too often, enthusiastic parents have been "turned off" by a professional's superior attitude or unrealistic demands. Professionals would do well to remember that parents and professionals have their own roles to play. When those individual roles are played in harmony with each other, the result is like a symphony that, though sounding like one voice, is made up of hundreds of instruments performing their own parts, yet complementing one another.

When teachers play the role of parent trainer, working with the parents of handicapped children, they must realize that their role is different from that of the teacher trainer or volunteer trainer. Teachers as parent trainers need to be sensitive to the vulnerabilities of parents. Sometimes parents have to be "pushed" to use structure consistently; yet the sensitive professional will understand the parents' difficulties in changing the behavior of their children. The parents must be guided, step-by-step, to the point where they are competent to treat their own children at home.

Parent training can be accomplished in individual parent-professional meetings or in group meetings. Group meetings are effective because didactic information can be given to several families at once. Also,. group meetings allow parents to get to know the parents of other autistic children. Thus a camaraderie, of sorts, is established.

At some point, usually when the parent has acquired basic behavior management skills, opportunities to work with the child under the parent trainer's supervision should be arranged. This can be accomplished either in the classroom or clinic or in the child's home. Teaching the parent to work with the child in the home has several advantages. One is that skills learned in school are more likely to generalize to the home if those skills are also taught in the home. The other advantage is that autistic children frequently exhibit different sets of behavior problems at home and at school. For example, at home, the child may throw tantrums to have needs met, but not throw tantrums at school. The same child may have toilet failures at school but be perfectly toilet trained at home. The teacher or parent trainer can more directly help parents deal with behavior problems in the home by "being there" to guide them through reinforcement and punishment procedures.

Substance and Strategies

Parent training should begin with information about autism. It is surprising how many parents are told by physicians that their child is autistic, yet are given little information about the disorder or what to expect for their child in the way of progress and prognosis. Explanations and descriptions of the disorder can help parents understand that there are other families going through the same thing. Knowledge about the disorder can help parents cope with a lifelong condition that will not go away, but that can be made easier to bear by instruction and training.

One of the most valuable tools that parents can receive from professionals is a strategy for managing behavior problems. The persistence of disruptive and inappropriate behaviors is one of the key factors that lead parents to place their autistic children in institutions (R. Baer, White, & Hinerman, 1982). The principles of behavior management (including reinforcement, various types of punishment, keeping track of behaviors, and analyzing progress) should be coordinated between school or clinic and home. Target behaviors and intervention procedures should be selected by parents and teachers together so that the intervention is carried out in the child's total environment.

Parents should be kept informed of every aspect of the child's educational program. Parents should also be encouraged and taught to work on selected goals with the child at home. This is especially critical for the autistic child's communication programs. If the child is being taught a nonspeech communication system, the parents and siblings must also learn the system and must provide opportunities for the child to use the system at home. Parents should be asked to provide vocabulary lists containing the child's favorite toys, places, foods, and so forth. The child can then be required to use these words (or signs) in order to gain access to favorite toys, foods, and other items.

THE HOME SETTING

Parents who can work with their children at home can provide the much needed one-to-one teaching ratio, thereby affording their children a greater opportunity to learn a new skill. Parent training programs can teach parents how to work with their children by teaching them to use the discrete-trial teaching format. Parents do not have to be perfect therapists; however, they do need to be able to decipher what effect their own behavior has on their child's behavior. When they have mastered this principle, they are on their way to becoming competent behavior managers and instructors.

The process of learning to handle one's own child objectively and consistently is long and often tedious. Parents sometimes want to give up. They feel it is too difficult, too demanding, too confining for the child. The parent trainer's job is to keep the goal in the parent's view and to remind them constantly that it *will* be worth it.

The following example illustrates the rewards of successful parent participation. When Jamie was four years old, his mother was told by a psychiatrist that he was autistic. Jamie's mother sent him to a special school where behavior modification was the therapy mode. By nature, Jamie's mother was reserved; she did not like to get involved. Besides, she could not bear to watch her son being taken to timeout or going through overcorrection. Jamie's teachers persuaded the mother to come into the classroom for one hour each week, just to observe.

After two months of "just watching," Jamie's mother began to ask questions about his therapy. She had also noticed a positive change in his behavior as long as he was in the classroom. She asked Jamie's teachers what she could do at home to achieve the same positive results.

After eight weeks of individual training (two hours each week), Jamie's mother began to work with Jamie in the classroom. She carried on the work at home; and Jamie did, indeed, make progress. Six months later, Jamie's mother was training another parent. A year later, she was at a parents' group meeting, where she was complimented by another parent on her zeal and precision in working with her autistic son. Jamie's mother replied, "There is so much for him to learn, and so little time. When I go to bed at night, I lie awake for hours thinking of things I want to teach him. I feel I shouldn't waste a minute. I want to wake him up in the middle of the night and work with him. There is just so much to do."

SUMMARY

Ensuring that autistic children reach their full potential involves every member of the children's environment. Studies have demonstrated that parental attitudes do not cause autism; rather, parents must be included as members of the educational team. Parents have the right and the responsibility to participate in the placement and development of goals for their autistic children. Parents cannot be expected to become therapists; yet they can, and should, be taught the skills necessary for managing their autistic children in the home. At the same time, parents can be valuable members of the educational team, since they have insight into their children's behavior and can often supplement classroom teaching.

The sensitive and perceptive teacher will be aware of parents' reluctance to become involved, but will develop ways to include them in every aspect of their child's education. Although the problems of having a handicapped child will never completely disappear, teachers can help parents find ways to cope with some of the problems and ways to change other problems.

References

American Psychiatric Association. *Diagnostic and statistical manual of mental disorders* (3rd ed.). Washington, D.C.: American Psychiatric Association, 1980.

Ando, H., Yoshimura, I., & Wakabayash, S. Effects of age on adaptive behavior levels in autistic children and mentally retarded children. *Journal of Autism and Developmental Disorders*, 1980, *10*, 123–184.

Archer, L.A. Blissymbolics—A nonverbal communication system. *Journal of Speech and Hearing Disorders*, 1977, *42*, 568–579.

Argyle, M. Non-verbal communication in human social interaction. In R.A. Hinde (Ed.), *Non-Vocal Communication*. London: Cambridge University Press, 1972.

Arick, J., & Krug, D. Autistic children: A study of learning characteristics and programming needs. *American Journal of Mental Deficiency*, 1978, *83*, 200–202.

Axelrod, S., Brantner, J.P., & Meddock, T.D. Overcorrection: A review and critical analysis. *Journal of Special Education*, 1978, *12*, 367–392.

Azrin, N.H., & Foxx, R.M. A rapid method of toilet training the institutionalized retarded. *Journal of Applied Behavior Analysis*, 1971, *4*, 89–99.

Azrin, N.H., Gottlieb, L., Hugart, L., Wesolowski, M.D., & Rahn, T. Eliminating self-injurious behavior by educational procedures. *Behavioral Research and Therapy*, 1975, *13*, 101–111.

Azrin, N.H., Kaplan, S.J., & Foxx, R.M. Autism reversal: Eliminating stereotyped self-stimulation of retarded individuals. *American Journal of Mental Deficiency*, 1973, *78*, 241–248.

Azrin, N.H., & Wesolowski, M.D. Eliminating habitual vomiting in a retarded adult by positive practice and self-correction. *Journal of Behavior Therapy and Experimental Psychiatry*, 1975, *6*, 145–148. (a)

Azrin, N.H., & Wesolowski, M.D. The use of positive practice to eliminate persistent floor sprawling by profoundly retarded persons. *Behavior Therapy*, 1975, *6*, 627–631. (b)

Baer, D., Peterson, R., & Sherman, J. The development of imitation by reinforcing behavioral similarity to a model. *Journal of Experimental Analysis of Behavior*, 1967, *10*, 405–416.

Baer, R., White, M.I., & Hinerman, P.S. *Factors influencing parents of autistic children to institutionalize their children.* Paper presented at the annual meeting of the National Society for Children and Adults with Autism, Omaha, Nebr., 1982.

171

Baker, B.L., Brightman, A.J., Heifetz, L.J., & Murphy, D.M. *Behavior problems.* Champaign, Ill.: Research Press, 1976.

Baker, L., Cantwell, D.P., Rutter, J., & Bartak, L. Language and autism. In E.R. Ritvo (Ed.), *Autism: Diagnosis, current research and management.* New York: Spectrum Publications, 1976.

Baldwin, V.L., Fredericks, H.D., & Brodsky, G. *"Isn't it time he outgrew this? or A training program for parents of retarded children.* Springfield, Ill.: Charles C Thomas, 1973.

Baltaxe, C., & Simmons, J.G. Language in childhood psychosis. *Journal of Speech and Hearing Disorders,* 1975, *40,* 439–458.

Baltaxe, C., & Simmons, J.G. Bedtime soliloquies and linguistic competence in autism. *Journal of Speech and Hearing Disorders,* 1977, *42,* 376–393.

Bandura, A. *Principles of behavior modification.* New York: Holt, Rinehart & Winston, 1969.

Barrera, R.D., Lobato-Barrera, D., & Sulzer-Azaroff, B. A stimulus treatment comparison of three expressive language training programs with a mute autistic child. *Journal of Autism and Developmental Disorders,* 1980, *10,* 21–37.

Bartak, L., & Rutter, M. The use of personal pronouns by autistic children. *Journal of Autism and Childhood Schizophrenia,* 1974, *4,* 217–222.

Bartolucci, G., & Albers, R.J. Deictic categories in the language of autistic children. *Journal of Autism and Childhood Schizophrenia,* 1974, *4,* 131–141.

Bartolucci, G., Pierce, S.J., Streiner, D., & Eppel, P.T. Phonological investigation of verbal autistic and mentally retarded subjects. *Journal of Autism and Childhood Schizophrenia,* 1976, *6,* 303–316.

Becker, W.C. *Parents are teachers.* Champaign, Ill.: Research Press, 1971.

Becker, W.C., Englemann, S., & Thomas, D.R. *Teaching: A course in applied psychology.* Chicago: Scientific Research Associates, 1971.

Benaroya, S., Wesley, S., Ogilvie, H., Klein, L.S., & Meany, M. Sign language and multisensory input training of children with communication and related developmental disorders. *Journal of Autism and Childhood Schizophrenia,* 1977, *7,* 23–32.

Bender, L. Childhood schizophrenia, a clinical study of one hundred schizophrenia. *American Journal of Orthopsychiatry,* 1947, *17,* 40–56.

Bernard-Opitz, V. Pragmatic analysis of the communication behavior of an autistic child. *Journal of Speech and Hearing Disorders,* 1982, *47,* 99–109.

Berry, M.F. *Teaching linguistically handicapped children.* Englewood Cliffs, N.J.: Prentice-Hall, 1980.

Bettelheim, B. *The empty fortress.* New York: Macmillan Publishing Co., 1967.

Bleuler, E. Autistic thinking. *American Journal of Insanity,* 1913, *69,* 873–886.

Bloom, L., & Lahey, M. *Language development and language disorders.* New York: John Wiley & Sons, 1978.

Bonvillian, J.D., & Nelson, K.E. Sign language acquisition in a mute autistic boy. *Journal of Speech and Hearing Disorders,* 1976, *41,* 339–347.

Bowerman, M. Semantic factors in the acquisition of rules for word use and sentence construction. In D.M. Morehead & A.E. Morehead (Eds.), *Normal and deficient child language.* Baltimore: University Park Press, 1976.

Bricker, W.A., & Bricker, D.D. An early language training strategy. In R.L. Schiefelbusch & L.L. Lloyd (Eds.), *Language perspectives: Acquisition, retardation, and intervention.* Baltimore: University Park Press, 1974.

Bricker, D.D., & Carlson, L. Issues in early language intervention. In R.L. Schiefelbusch & D.D. Bricker (Eds.), *Early language: Acquisition and intervention*. Baltimore: University Park Press, 1981.

Bucher, B., & Lovaas, O.I. Use of aversive stimulation in behavior modification. In M.R. Jones (Ed.), *Miami symposium on the prediction of behavior: Aversive stimulation*. Coral Gables, Fla.: University of Miami Press, 1968.

Cantwell, D.P., Baker, L., & Rutter, M. Families of autistic and dysphasic children. II: Mother's speech to the children. *Journal of Autism and Childhood Schizophrenia*, 1977, *7*, 313; 327.

Carlson, F. A format for selecting vocabulary for the nonspeaking child. *Language, Speech, and Hearing Services in Schools*, 1981, *12*, 240–245.

Carr, E.G. Generalization of treatment effects following educational intervention with autistic children and youth. In B. Wilcox & A. Thompson (Eds.), *Critical issues in educating autistic children and youth*. Washington, D.C.: U.S. Department of Education, Office of Special Education, 1980.

Carr, E.G., Binkoff, J.A., Kologinsky, E., & Eddy, M. Acquisition of sign language by autistic children: I. Expressive labeling. *Journal of Applied Behavior Analysis*, 1978, *11*, 489–501.

Carr, J. The severely retarded autistic child. In L. Wing (Ed.), *Early childhood autism*. New York: Pergamon Press, 1976.

Carrier, J.K. Application of functional analysis and a nonspeech response mode to teaching language. In L.V. McReynolds (Ed.), *Developing systematic procedures for training children's language, American Speech and Hearing Association Monograph*, 1974, (No. 18), 47–95.

Carrier, J.K., & Peak, T. *Non-speech language initiation program*. Lawrence, Kans.: H & H Enterprises, 1975.

Casey, L.O. Development of communicative behavior in autistic children: A parent program using manual signs. *Journal of Autism and Childhood Schizophrenia*, 1978, *8*, 45–59.

Chess, S. Follow-up report on autism in congenital rubella. *Journal of Autism and Childhood Schizophrenia*, 1977, *7*, 69–81.

Churchill, D.W. The relation of infantile autism and early childhood schizophrenia to developmental language disorders of childhood. *Journal of Autism and Childhood Schizophrenia*, 1972, *2*, 182–197.

Churchill, D.W. Language: The problem beyond conditioning. In M. Rutter & E. Schopler (Eds.), *Autism: A reappraisal of concepts and treatment*. New York: Plenum Press, 1978.

Clark, C.R., Davies, C.O., & Woodcock, R.N. *Standard rebus dictionary*. Circle Pines, Minn.: American Guidance Service, 1974.

Clark, P., & Rutter, M. Compliance and resistance in autistic children. *Journal of Autism and Childhood Schizophrenia*, 1977, *7*, 33–48.

Clark, P., & Rutter, M. Autistic children's responses to structure and to interpersonal demands. *Journal of Autism and Developmental Disorders*, 1981, *11*, 201–217.

Cohen, D.J., Young, J.G., Lowe, T.L., & Harcherik, D. Thyroid hormone in autistic children. *Journal of Autism and Developmental Disorders*, 1980, *10*, 445–449.

Cohen, M. *The development of language behavior in an autistic child using a total communication approach*. Paper presented at the annual meeting of the Council for Exceptional Children, Dallas, 1979.

Cole, M.L., & Cole, J.T. *Effective intervention with the language impaired child.* Rockville, Md.: Aspen Systems Corp., 1981.

Coleman, M. Serotonin and central nervous system syndromes of childhood. *Journal of Autism and Childhood Schizophrenia,* 1973, *3,* 27–35.

Coleman, M. *New research findings and concepts in autism.* Paper presented at the annual meeting of the National Society for Children and Adults with Autism, Washington, D.C., 1980.

Condon, W.S. Multiple response to sound in dysfunctional children. *Journal of Autism and Childhood Schizophrenia,* 1975, *5,* 37–56.

Costello, J.M. Programmed instruction. *Journal of Speech and Hearing Disorders,* 1977, *42,* 3–28.

Courtright, J.A., & Courtright, I.C. Imitation modeling as a language intervention strategy: The effects of two mediating variables. *Journal of Speech and Hearing Research,* 1979, *22,* 389–402.

Creak, M. Schizophrenia syndrome in childhood. Progress report (April, 1961) of a working party. *British Medical Journal,* 1961, *2,* 889–890.

Creak, M. Reflections on communication and autistic children. *Journal of Autism and Childhood Schizophrenia,* 1972, *2,* 1–8.

Creedon, M. *Language development in nonverbal autistic children using a simultaneous communication system.* Paper presented at the meeting of the Society for Research in Child Development, Philadelphia, 1973.

Cromer, R.F. Developmental language disorders: Cognitive processes, semantics, pragmatics, phonology, and syntax. *Journal of Autism and Developmental Disabilities,* 1981, *11,* 57–74.

Cunningham, M., & Dixon, C. A study of the language of an autistic child. *Journal of Child Psychology and Psychiatry,* 1961, *2,* 193–202.

Curcio, F., & Piserchia, E.A. Pantomimic representation in psychotic children. *Journal of Autism and Childhood Schizophrenia,* 1978, *8,* 181–189.

Czyzewski, M.J., Barrera, R.D., & Sulzer-Azaroff, B. An abbreviated overcorrection program to reduce self-stimulatory behaviors. *Journal of Behavior Therapy and Experimental Psychiatry,* 1982, *13,* 55–62.

Dale, P.S. *Language development: Structure and function.* Hinsdale, Ill.: Dryden Press, 1972.

Dalgeish, B. Cognitive processing and linguistic reference in autistic children. *Journal of Autism and Childhood Schizophrenia,* 1975, *5,* 353–361.

Daniloff, J.K., & Shafer, A. A gestural communication program for severely and profoundly handicapped children. *Language, Speech, and Hearing Services in School,* 1981, *12,* 258–267.

Dawson, G., Warrenburg, S., & Fuller, P. Cerebral lateralization in individuals diagnosed as autistic in early childhood. *Brain and Language,* 1982, *15,* 353–368.

DeLong, G.R. A neuropsychologic interpretation of infantile autism. In M. Rutter & E. Schopler (Eds.), *Autism: A reappraisal of concepts and treatment.* New York: Plenum Press, 1978.

DeMyer, M.K. Perceptual limitations in autistic children and their relation to social and intellectual deficits. In M. Rutter (Ed.), *Infantile autism: Concepts, characteristics, and treatment.* London: Churchill Livingston, 1971.

DeMyer, M.K. *Parents and children in autism.* Washington, D.C.: V.H. Winston & Sons, 1979.

DeMyer, M.K., Alpern, G.D., Barton, S., DeMyer, W.E., Churchill, D.W., Hingtgen, J.N., Bryson, C.Q., Pontius, W., & Kimberlin, C. Imitation in autistic, early schizophrenia, and non-psychotic subnormal children. *Journal of Autism and Childhood Schizophrenia,* 1972, *2,* 264–287.

DeMyer, M.K., Barton, S., DeMyer, W.E., Norton, J.A., Allen, J., & Steele, R. Prognosis in autism: A follow-up study. *Journal of Autism and Childhood Schizophrenia,* 1973, *3,* 199–246.

DeMyer, M.K., Norton, J.A., & Barton, S. Social and adaptive behaviors of autistic children as measured in a structured psychiatric interview. In D.W. Churchill, G.D. Alpern, & M.K. DeMyer (Eds.), *Infantile autism.* Springfield, Ill.: Charles C Thomas, 1971.

DesLauriers, A.M. Play, symbols, and the development of language. In M. Rutter & E. Schopler (Eds.), *Autism: A reappraisal of concepts and treatment.* New York: Plenum Press, 1978.

Despert, L. *Schizophrenia in children.* New York: Robert Brunner, 1968.

Doke, L.A., & Epstein, L.H. Oral overcorrection: Side effects of extended applications. *Journal of Experimental Child Psychology,* 1975, *20,* 496–511.

Donnellan, A.M. An educational perspective of autism: Implications for curriculum development and personnel development. In B. Wilcox & A. Thompson (Eds.), *Critical issues in educating autistic children and youth.* Washington, D.C.: U.S. Department of Education, Office of Special Education, 1980.

Donnellan, A.M., Gossage, L.D., LaVigna, G.W., Schuler, A.L., & Traphagen, J.D. *Teaching makes a difference.* Sacramento: California State Department of Education, 1977.

Dores, P.A., & Carr, E.G. *Sign language comprehension by autistic children following simultaneous communication training.* Paper presented at the annual meeting of the American Psychological Association, New York, 1979.

Eisenberg, L. The autistic child in adolescence. *American Journal of Psychiatry,* 1956, *112,* 607–612.

Eisenson, J. *Aphasia in children.* New York: Harper & Row, 1972.

Epstein, L.H., Doke, L.A., Sajwaj, T.E., Sorrell, S., & Rimmer, B. Generality and side effects of overcorrection. *Journal of Applied Behavior Analysis,* 1974, *7,* 386–390.

Etemad, J.G., Szurek, S.A., Yeager, C.L., & Schulkin, F.R. Evaluation of EEG findings in a group of psychotic children. In S.A. Szurek & I.N. Berlin (Eds.), *Clinical studies in childhood psychosis.* New York: Brunner/Mazel, 1973.

Everard, P. *Involuntary strangers.* London: John Clare Books, 1980.

Fay, W., & Schuler, A.L. *Emerging language in autistic children.* Baltimore: University Park Press, 1980.

Fish, B. Biological disorders in infants at risk for schizophrenia. In E.R. Ritvo (Ed.), *Autism: Diagnosis, current research, and management.* New York: Spectrum Publications, 1976. (a)

Fish, B. Pharmacotherapy for autistic and schizophrenic children. In E.R. Ritvo (Ed.), *Autism: Diagnosis, current research, and management.* New York: Spectrum Publications, 1976. (b)

Flaharty, R. Educational approaches at the NPI school: Preschool assessment. In E.R. Ritvo (Ed.), *Autism: Diagnosis, current research, and management.* New York: Spectrum Publications, 1976.

Foxx, R.M. Attention training: The use of overcorrection avoidance to increase the eye contact of autistic and retarded children. *Journal of Applied Behavior Analysis,* 1977, *10,* 489–499.

Foxx, R.M. *Effective behavioral programming.* Champaign, Ill.: Research Press, 1980. (a)

Foxx, R.M. *Working with the self-abusive individual.* Paper presented at the meeting of the National Society for Children and Adults with Autism, 1980. (b)

Foxx, R.M., & Azrin, N.H. Restitution: A method of eliminating aggressive-disruptive behavior of mentally retarded and brain damaged patients. *Behavior Research and Therapy,* 1972, *10,* 15–27.

Foxx, R.M., & Azrin, N.H. The elimination of autistic self-stimulatory behavior by overcorrection. *Journal of Applied Behavior Analysis,* 1973, *6,* 1–14. (a)

Foxx, R.M., & Azrin, N.H. *Toilet training the retarded.* Champaign, Ill.: Research Press, 1973. (b)

Frankel, F., Tymchuk, A.J., & Simmons, J.Q. Operant analysis and intervention with autistic children: Implications of current research. In E.R. Ritvo (Ed.), *Autism: Diagnosis, current research, and management.* New York: Spectrum Publications, 1976.

Freeman, B.J., Graham, V., & Ritvo, E.R. Reduction of self-destructive behavior by overcorrection. *Psychological Reports,* 1975, *37,* 446.

Freeman, B.J., & Ritvo, E.R. Parents as professionals. In E.R. Ritvo (Ed.), *Autism: Diagnosis, current research, and management.* New York: Spectrum Publications, 1976.

Freeman, B.J., Ritvo, E.R., & Miller, R. An operant procedure to teach an echolalic, autistic child to answer questions appropriately. *Journal of Autism and Childhood Schizophrenia,* 1975, *5,* 169–176.

Freeman, B.J., Schroth, P., Ritvo, E.R., Guthrie, D., & Wake, L. The Behavior Observation Scale for Autism (BOS): Initial results of factor analysis. *Journal of Autism and Developmental Disorders,* 1980, *11,* 343–346.

Fulwiler, R.L., & Fouts, R.S. Acquisition of American sign language by a noncommunicating autistic child. *Journal of Autism and Childhood Schizophrenia,* 1976, *6,* 43–51.

Gallaudet, T.H. On the natural language of signs, and its value and uses in the instruction of the deaf and dumb. In R.L. Schiefelbusch (Ed.), *Nonspeech language and communication: Analysis and intervention.* Baltimore: University Park Press, 1980.

Gaylord-Ross, R. A decision model for the treatment of aberrant behavior in applied settings. In W. Sailor, B. Wilcox, & L. Brown (Eds.), *Methods of instruction for severely handicapped students.* Baltimore: University Park Press, 1980.

Gelfand, D.M., & Hartmann, D.P. *Child behavior: Analysis and therapy.* New York: Pergamon Press, 1975.

Goetz, L., Schuler, A., & Sailor, W. Teaching functional speech to the severely handicapped: Current issues. *Journal of Autism and Developmental Disorders,* 1979, *9,* 325–343.

Goldfarb, W., Goldfarb, N., Braunstein, P., & Scholl, H. Speech and language faults of schizophrenic children. *Journal of Autism and Childhood Schizophrenia,* 1972, *2,* 219–223.

Goldfarb, W., Yadkovitz, E., & Goldfarb, N. Verbal symbols to designate objects: An experimental study of communication in mothers of schizophrenic children. *Journal of Autism and Childhood Schizophrenia,* 1973, *3,* 281–298.

Goldman, P.S. Development and plasticity of frontal association cortex in the infrahuman primate. In C.L. Ludlow & M.E. Doran-Quine (Eds.), *The neurological bases of language disorders in children: Methods and directions for research* (NINCDS Monograph No. 22). Bethesda, Md.: U.S. Department of Health, Education, and Welfare, 1979.

Gray, B., & Ryan, B. *A language program for the nonlanguage child*. Champaign, Ill.: Research Press, 1973.

Gross, A.M., Berler, E.S., & Drabman, R.S. Reduction of aggressive behavior in a retarded boy using a water squirt. *Journal of Behavior Therapy and Experimental Psychiatry*, 1982, *13*, 95–98.

Guess, D., Sailor, W., & Baer, D.M. To teach language to retarded children. In R.L. Schiefelbusch & L.L. Lloyd (Eds.), *Language perspectives: Acquisition, retardation, and intervention*. Baltimore: University Park Press, 1974.

Gustason, G., Pfetzing, D., & Zawolkow, E. *Signing exact English*. Los Alamitos, Calif.: Modern Signs Press, 1980.

Handleman, J.S. Transfer of verbal response across instructional settings by autistic-type children. *Journal of Speech and Hearing Disorders*, 1981, *46*, 69–79.

Handleman, J.S., & Harris, S.L. Generalization from school to home with autistic children. *Journal of Autism and Developmental Disorders*, 1980, *10*, 323–333.

Harper, J., & Williams, S. Age and type of onset as critical variables in early infantile autism. *Journal of Autism and Childhood Schizophrenia*, 1975, *5*, 25–36.

Harris, S.L. Teaching language to nonverbal children—with emphasis on problems of generalization. *Psychological Bulletin*, 1975, *82*, 565–580.

Harris, S.L., & Romanczyk, R.G. Treating self-injurious behavior of a retarded child by overcorrection. *Behavior Therapy*, 1976, *7*, 235–239.

Hassibi, M., & Breuer, H. *Disordered thinking and communication in children*. New York: Plenum Press, 1980.

Hauser, S.L., DeLong, G.R., & Rosman, N.P. Pneumographic findings in the infantile autism syndrome. *Brain*, 1975, *98*, 667–688.

Hermelin, B. Rules and language. In M. Rutter (Ed.), *Infantile autism: Concepts, characteristics, and treatment*. London: Churchill Livingston, 1971.

Hermelin, B. Images and language. In M. Rutter & E. Schopler (Eds.), *Autism: A reappraisal of concepts and treatment*. New York: Plenum Press, 1978.

Hinerman, P.S., Jenson, W.R., Walker, G.R., & Petersen, P.B. Positive practice overcorrection combined with additional procedures to teach signed words to an autistic child. *Journal of Autism and Developmental Disorders*, 1982, *12*, 253–263.

Hinerman, P.S., Walker, G.R., & Jenson, W.R. *Simultaneous communication used as a language mediator for an autistic boy*. Paper presented at the meeting of the American Speech/Language and Hearing Association, Atlanta, 1979.

Hollis, J.H., & Carrier, J.K. Intervention strategies for nonspeech children. In R.L. Schiefelbusch (Ed.), *Nonspeech language and communication: Analysis and intervention*. Baltimore: University Park Press, 1978.

Horner, R.D., & Barton, E.S. Operant techniques in the analysis and modification of self-injurious behavior: A review. *Behavior Research of Severe Developmental Disabilities*, 1980, *1*, 61–191.

Howlin, P. The assessment of social behavior. In M. Rutter & E. Schopler (Eds.), *Autism: A reappraisal of concepts and treatment*. New York: Plenum Press, 1978.

Hurtig, R., Ensrud, S., & Tomblin, J.B. The communicative function of question production in autistic children. *Journal of Autism and Developmental Disorders*, 1982, *12*, 57–69.

Israel, M. Educational approaches at the Behavior Research Institute, Providence, Rhode Island. In E.R. Ritvo (Ed.), *Autism: Diagnosis, current research, and management.* New York: Spectrum Publications, 1976.

Jackson, M.J., & Garrod, P.J. Plasma zinc, copper, and amino acid levels in the blood of autistic children. *Journal of Autism and Childhood Schizophrenia,* 1978, *8,* 203–208.

Kamhi, A.G. Nonlinguistic symbolic and conceptual abilities of language-impaired and normally developing children. *Journal of Speech and Hearing Research,* 1981, *24,* 446–453.

Kanner, L. Autistic disturbance of affective contact. *Nervous Child,* 1943, *2,* 242–250.

Kanner, L. Irrelevant and metaphorical language in early infantile autism. *American Journal of Psychiatry,* 1946, *103,* 242–246.

Kanner, L. *Child psychiatry.* Springfield, Ill.: Charles C Thomas, 1957. (Originally published in 1935.)

Kanner, L. The birth of early infantile autism. *Journal of Autism and Childhood Schizophrenia,* 1973, *3,* 93–95.

Kelly, J.A., & Drabman, R.S. Overcorrection: An effective procedure that failed. *Journal of Clinical Child Psychology,* 1977, *6,* 38–40.

Kent, L. *Language acquisition program for the severely retarded.* Champaign, Ill.: Research Press, 1974.

Kiernan, C. A strategy for research on the use of nonvocal systems of communication. *Journal of Autism and Developmental Disorders,* 1981, *11,* 139–151.

Koegel, R.L., & Covert, A. The relationship of self-stimulation to learning in autistic children. *Journal of Applied Behavior Analysis,* 1972, *5,* 381–387.

Koegel, R.L., Dunlap, G., & Dyer, K. Intertrial interval duration and learning in autistic children. *Journal of Applied Behavior Analysis,* 1980, *13,* 91–99.

Koegel, R.L., & Egel, A.L. Motivating autistic children. *Journal of Abnormal Child Psychology,* 1979, *88,* 418–426.

Koegel, R.L., Egel, A.L., & Dunlap, G. Learning characteristics of autistic children. In W. Sailor, B. Wilcox, & L. Brown (Eds.), *Methods of instruction for severely handicapped students.* Baltimore: Paul H. Brooks, 1980.

Koegel, R.L., Russo, D.C., & Rincover, A. Assessing and training teachers in the generalized use of behavior modification with autistic children. *Journal of Applied Behavior Analysis,* 1977, *10,* 197–205.

Koegel, R.L., & Williams, J.A. Direct versus indirect response-reinforcer relationships in teaching autistic children. *Journal of Abnormal Child Psychology,* 1980, *8,* 537–547.

Konstantareas, M.M., Hunter, D., & Sloman, L. Training a blind autistic child to communicate through signs. *Journal of Autism and Developmental Disorders,* 1982, *12,* 1–12.

Konstantareas, M.M., Webster, C.D., & Oxman, J. An alternative to speech training: Simultaneous communication. In C.D. Webster, M.M. Konstantareas, J. Oxman, & J.E. Mack (Eds.), *Autism: New directions in research and education.* New York: Pergamon Press, 1980.

Krug, D.A., Arick, J.R., & Almond, P.J. *Autism Screening Instrument for Educational Planning.* Portland, Oreg.: ASIEP Education Company, 1980.

Krug, D.A., Arick, J.R., Scanlon, C., Almond, P.J., Rosenblum, J.F., & Border, M. Evaluation of a program of systematic instructional procedures for preverbal autistic children. *Improving Human Performance Quarterly,* 1979, *8,* 29–41.

Krug, D.A., Rosenblum, J.F., Almond, P.J., & Arick, J.R. *Autistic and severely handicapped in the classroom: Assessment, behavior management, and communication training.* Portland, Oreg.: ASIEP Education Company, 1981.

Krumboltz, J.D., & Krumboltz, H.B. *Changing children's behavior.* Englewood Cliffs, N.J.: Prentice-Hall, 1972.

Kyne, J. The evolving parent-professional relationship. In B. Wilcox & A. Thompson (Eds.), *Critical issues in educating autistic children and youth.* Washington, D.C.: National Society for Children and Adults with Autism, 1980.

Kysela, G., Hillyard, A., McDonald, L., & Ahlsten-Taylor, J. Early intervention: Design and evaluation. In R.L. Schiefelbusch & D.D. Bricker (Eds.), *Early language: Acquisition and intervention.* Baltimore: University Park Press, 1981.

Lamendella, J.T. The limbic system in human communication. In H. Whitaker & H.A. Whitaker (Eds.), *Studies in neurolinguistics.* New York: Academic Press, 1977.

Langacker, R. *Language and its structure.* New York: Harcourt Brace Jovanovich, 1967.

LaVigna, G.W. Communication training in mute autistic adolescents using the written word. *Journal of Autism and Childhood Schizophrenia,* 1977, *7,* 135–149.

Lelord, G., Muh, J.P., Barthelemy, G., Martineau, J., Garreau, G., & Callaway, E. Effects of pyridoxine and magnesium on autistic symptoms: Initial observations. *Journal of Autism and Developmental Disorders,* 1981, *11,* 219–230.

Lennox, C., Callias, M., & Rutter, M. Cognitive characteristics of parents of autistic children. *Journal of Autism and Childhood Schizophrenia,* 1977, *7,* 243–261.

Links, P.S. Minor physical anomalies in childhood autism: Part II. Their relationship to maternal age. *Journal of Autism and Developmental Disorders,* 1980, *10,* 287–297.

Links, P.S., Stockwell, M., Abichandani, F., & Simeon, J. Minor physical anomalies in childhood autism. Part I: Their relationship to pre- and perinatal complications. *Journal of Autism and Developmental Disorders,* 1980, *10,* 273–285.

Litrownik, A.J., McInnis, E.T., Wetzel-Pritchard, A.M., & Filipelli, D.L. Restricted stimulus control and inferred attentional deficits in autistic and retarded children. *Journal of Abnormal Psychology,* 1978, *87,* 554–562.

Lord, C., & O'Neill, P.J. A developmental-behavior model for the prescriptive evaluation of autistic and severely socially impaired children. In B. Wilcox & A. Thompson (Eds.), *Critical issues in educating autistic children and youth.* Washington, D.C.: U.S. Department of Education, Office of Education, 1980.

Lotter, V. Factors related to outcome in autistic children. *Journal of Autism and Childhood Schizophrenia,* 1974, *4,* 263–277.

Lovaas, O.I. A program for the establishment of speech in psychotic children. In H.N. Sloane & B.D. MacAulay (Eds.), *Operant procedures in remedial speech and language training.* Boston: Houghton Mifflin Co., 1968.

Lovaas, O.I. *The autistic child: Language development through behavior modification.* New York: Irvington Publishers, 1977.

Lovaas, O.I. Parents as therapists. In M. Rutter & E. Schopler (Eds.), *Autism: A reappraisal of concepts and treatment.* New York: Plenum Press, 1978.

Lovaas, O.I. *Teaching developmentally disabled children: The me book.* Baltimore: University Park Press, 1981.

Lovaas, O.I., Berberich, J.P., Perloff, B.F., & Schaeffer, B. Acquisition of imitative speech by schizophrenic children. *Science,* 1966, *151,* 705–707.

Lovaas, O.I., Koegel, R.L., & Schreibman, L. Stimulus overselectivity in autism: A review of research. *Psychological Bulletin,* 1979, *6,* 1236–1254.

Lovaas, O.I., Schaeffer, B., & Simmons, J.Q. Experimental studies in childhood schizophrenia: Building social behavior by use of electric shock. *Journal of Experimental Studies in Personality,* 1965, *1,* 99–109.

Lovaas, O.I., Schreibman, L., & Koegel, R.L. A behavior modification approach to the treatment of autistic children. *Journal of Autism and Childhood Schizophrenia,* 1974, *4,* 111–129.

Lovaas, O.I., Schreibman, L., Koegel, R.L., & Rehm, R. Selective responding by autistic children to multiple sensory input. *Journal of Abnormal Psychology,* 1971, *77,* 211–222.

Lowell, M. Audiological assessment. In E.R. Ritvo (Ed.), *Autism: Diagnosis, current research and management.* New York: Spectrum Publications, 1976.

Lucas, E.V. *Semantic and pragmatic language disorders.* Rockville, Md.: Aspen Systems Corp., 1980.

Lyons, J. Human Language. In R.A. Hinde (Ed.), *Non-vocal communication.* London: Cambridge University Press, 1972.

MacKay, D.M. Formal analysis of communication processes. In R.A. Hinde (Ed.), *Non-vocal communication.* London: Cambridge University Press, 1972.

Mager, R. *Preparing instructional objectives.* Belmont, Calif.: Feron Publishers, 1975.

Mahler, M.S. On child psychosis and schizophrenia, autistic and symbiotic infantile psychosis. *Psychoanalytic Study of the Child,* 1952, *7,* 286–305.

Marcus, L.M. Developmental assessment as a basis for planning educational programs for autistic children. *Behavioral Disorders,* 1978, *3,* 219–226.

McDonald, E.T. Design and application of communication boards. In G.C. Vanderheiden & K. Grilley (Eds.), *Non-vocal communication techniques and aids for the severely physically handicapped.* Baltimore: University Park Press, 1975. (a)

McDonald, E.T. Identification of children at risk. In G.C. Vanderheiden & K. Grilley (Eds.) *Non-vocal communication techniques and aids for the severely physically handicapped.* Baltimore: University Park Press, 1975. (b)

McDonald, E.T. Language foundations. In G.C. Vanderheiden & K. Grilley (Eds.), *Non-vocal communication techniques and aids for the severely physically handicapped.* Baltimore: University Park Press, 1975. (c).

McDonald, E.T. *Teaching and using blissymbolics.* Toronto: Blissymbolics Communication Institute, 1980.

McGowan, M., & Webster, C.D. Autism and the Condon effect: An elaboration of the evidence with additional hypotheses and suggestions for educational programs. In C.D. Webster, M.M. Konstantareas, J. Oxman, & J.E. Mack (Eds.), *Autism: New directions in research and education.* New York: Pergamon Press, 1980.

McNaughton, S. Bliss symbols—An alternative symbol system for the non-vocal pre-reading child. In G.C. Vanderheiden & K. Grilley (Eds.), *Non-vocal communication techniques and aids for the severely physically handicapped.* Baltimore: University Park Press, 1975.

Menolascino, F.J., & Eyde, D.R. Biophysical bases of autism. *Behavioral Disorders,* 1979, *5,* 41–47.

Menyuk, P. The bases of language acquisition: Some questions. *Journal of Autism and Childhood Schizophrenia,* 1974, *4,* 325–345.

Menyuk, P. Language: What's wrong and why. In M. Rutter & E. Schopler (Eds.), *Autism: A reappraisal of concepts and treatment.* New York: Plenum Press, 1978.

Metcalf, A.W. An experience with the Rimland checklist for autism. In S.A. Szurek & I.R. Berlin (Eds.), *Clinical studies in childhood psychosis*. New York: Brunner/Mazel, 1973.

Miller, A.M., & Miller, E.E. Cognitive developmental training with elevated boards and sign language. *Journal of Autism and Childhood Schizophrenia*, 1973, *3*, 65–85.

Miller, J.F. *Assessing language production in children*. Baltimore: University Park Press, 1981.

Miller, J.F., & Yoder, D.E. An ontogenetic language teaching strategy for retarded children. In R.L. Schiefelbusch & L.L. Lloyd (Eds.), *Language perspectives: Acquisition, retardation, and intervention*. Baltimore: University Park Press, 1974.

Moores, D.F. American sign language. In R.L. Schiefelbusch (Ed.), *Nonspeech language and communication: Analysis and intervention*. Baltimore: University Park Press, 1980.

Moores, D.F. Issues in the modification of American sign language for instructional purposes. *Journal of Autism and Developmental Disorders*, 1981, *11*, 153–162.

Morrison, D., Miller, D., & Mejia, B. Comprehension and negation of verbal communication in autistic children. In S.A. Szurek & I.R. Berlin (Eds.), *Clinical studies in childhood psychosis*. New York: Brunner/Mazel, 1973.

Murdock, J.Y., & Hartmann, B.V. *A language development program: Imitative gestures to basic syntactic structures*. Salt Lake City, Utah: Work Making Productions, 1975.

National Society for Children and Adults with Autism. *Fact Sheet*. Washington, D.C.: National Institutes of Health, Department of Health and Human Services, 1980.

Needleman, R., Ritvo, E.R., & Freeman, B.J. Objectively define linguistic parameters in children with autism and other developmental disabilities. *Journal of Autism and Developmental Disorders*, 1980, *10*, 389–398.

Newsom, C., & Rincover, A. Autism. In E.J. Mash & L.G. Terdal (Eds.), *Behavioral assessment of childhood disorders*. New York: Guilford Press, 1981.

Ney, P.G. Effect of contingent and non-contingent reinforcement on the behavior of an autistic child. *Journal of Autism and Childhood Schizophrenia*, 1973, *3*, 115–127.

Nober, E.H., & Simmons, J.Q. Comparison of auditory stimulus processing in normal and autistic adolescents. *Journal of Autism and Developmental Disorders*, 1981, *11*, 175–189.

O'Conner, N. Visual perception in autistic children. In M . Rutter (Ed.), *Infantile autism: Concepts, characteristics and treatment*. London: Churchill Livingston, 1971.

O'Dell, S.L., Blackwell, L.J., Larcen, S.W., & Hogan, J.L. Competency-based training for severely behaviorally handicapped children and their parents. *Journal of Autism and Childhood Schizophrenia*, 1977, *7*, 231–242.

Ornitz, E.M. The modulation of sensory input and motor output in autistic children. *Journal of Autism and Childhood Schizophrenia*, 1974, *4*, 197–215.

Ornitz, E.M. Neurophysiologic studies. In M. Rutter & E. Schopler (Eds.), *Autism: A reappraisal of concepts and treatment*. New York: Plenum Press, 1978.

Ornitz, E.M., Guthrie, D., & Farley, A.H. The early development of autistic children. *Journal of Autism and Childhood Schizophrenia*, 1977, *7*, 207–229.

Ornitz, E.M., & Ritvo, E.R. Medical assessment. In E.R. Ritvo (Ed.), *Autism: Diagnosis, current research and management*. New York: Spectrum Publications, 1976.

Ornitz, E.M., Tanguay, P.E., Lee, J.C.M., Ritvo, E.R., Silvertsen, B., & Wilson, C. The effect of stimulus interval on the auditory evoked response during sleep in autistic children. *Journal of Autism and Childhood Schizophrenia*, 1972, *2*, 140–150.

Paccia, J., & Curcio, F. Language processing and forms of immediate echolalia in autistic children. *Journal of Speech and Hearing Research*, 1982, *25*, 42–47.

Palkovitz, R.J., & Wiesenfeld, R.J. Differential autonomic responses of autistic and normal children. *Journal of Autism and Developmental Disorders*, 1980, *10*, 347–360.

Paluszny, M.J. *Autism: A practical guide for parents and professionals.* Syracuse, N.Y.: Syracuse University Press, 1979.

Parry, J.K., & Brandt, L.J. *Language level and behavioral disturbances in autistic children.* Paper presented at the meeting of the International Conference on Autism, Boston, 1981.

Patterson, G.R. *Living with children.* Champaign, Ill.: Research Press, 1971.

Petretic, P.A., & Tweney, R.D. Does comprehension precede production? The development of children's responses to telegraphic sentences of varying grammatical adequacy. *Journal of Child Language*, 1977, *4*, 201–209.

Pierce, S., & Bartolucci, G. A syntactic investigation of verbal autistic, mentally retarded, and normal children. *Journal of Autism and Childhood Schizophrenia*, 1977, *7*, 121–134.

Popovitch, D., & Laham, S.L. (Eds.). *The adaptive behavior curriculum* (Vol. 1). Baltimore: Paul H. Brooks, 1981.

Premack, D. A functional analysis of language. *Journal of Experimental Analysis of Behavior*, 1970, *14*, 107–125.

Prior, M.R. Cognitive abilities and disabilities in infantile autism. *Journal of Abnormal Psychology*, 1979, *9*, 357–380.

Prizant, B.M. Speech-language pathologists and autistic children: What is our role? *American Speech-Language-Hearing Association*, 1982, *24*, 463–468.

Prizant, B.M., & Duchan, J.F. The foundation of immediate echolalia in autistic children. *Journal of Speech and Hearing Disorders*, 1981, *46*, 241–249.

Rank, B. Adaptation of the psychoanalytic technique for the treatment of young children with atypical development. *American Journal of Orthopsychiatry*, 1949, *19*, 130–139.

Rees, N.S. Imitation and language development. *Journal of Speech and Hearing Disorders*, 1975, *40*, 339–350.

Rees, S.C., & Taylor, A. Prognostic antecedents and outcome in a follow-up study of children with a diagnosis of childhood psychosis. *Journal of Autism and Childhood Schizophrenia*, 1975, *5*, 309–322.

Reese, E.P. *The analysis of human operant behavior.* Dubuque, Iowa: William C. Brown, 1966.

Reynolds, B., Newsom, C.D., & Lovaas, O.I. Auditory overselectivity in autistic children. *Journal of Abnormal Child Psychology*, 1974, *2*, 253–264.

Rice, M. *Cognition to language: Categories, word meanings, and training.* Baltimore: University Park Press, 1980.

Richer, J. The partial noncommunication of culture to autistic children—an application of human ethology. In M. Rutter & E. Schopler (Eds.), *Autism: A reappraisal of concepts and treatment.* New York: Plenum Press, 1978.

Ricks, D.M., & Wing, L. Language, communication, and the use of symbols in normal and autistic children. *Journal of Autism and Childhood Schizophrenia*, 1975, *5*, 191–221.

Rimland, B. *Infantile autism.* Englewood Cliffs, N.J.: Prentice-Hall, 1964.

Rimland, B. The differentiation of childhood psychosis: An analysis of checklists for 2,218 psychotic children. *Journal of Autism and Childhood Schizophrenia*, 1971, *1*, 161–174.

Rimland, B. Psychological treatment versus megavitamin therapy. In V. Binder, A. Binder, & B. Rimland (Eds.), *Modern therapies.* Englewood Cliffs, N.J.: Prentice-Hall, 1976.

Rimland, B. *Update research on the use of* B_{15}. Paper presented at the annual meeting of the National Society for Autistic Children, San Jose, Calif., 1979.

Rincover, A. Variables affecting stimulus fading and discriminative responding in psychotic children. *Journal of Abnormal Psychology*, 1978, *87*, 541–553.

Risley, T.R. The effects and side-effects of punishing the autistic behaviors of a deviant child. *Journal of Applied Behavior Analysis*, 1968, *1*, 21–34.

Ritvo, E.R. Autism: From adjective to noun. In E.R. Ritvo (Ed.), *Autism: Diagnosis, current research, and management*. New York: Spectrum Publications, 1976.

Roberts, P., Iwata, B.A., McSween, T.E., & Desmond, E.F. An analysis of overcorrection movements. *American Journal of Mental Deficiency*, 1979, *83*, 588–594.

Robinson, E., Hughes, H., Wilson, D., Lahey, B.B., & Haynes, S. *Modification of stereotyped behaviors of "autistic" children through response contingent water squirts*. Paper presented at the annual meeting of the Association for the Advancement of Behavior Therapy, Chicago, 1974.

Rodgon, M.M., Jankowski, W., & Alenskas, L. A multifunctional approach to single-word usage. *Journal of Child Language*, 1977, *4*, 23–43.

Rodnight, R. Biochemical strategies and concepts. In M. Rutter & E. Schopler (Eds.), *Autism: A reappraisal of concepts and treatment*. New York: Plenum Press, 1978.

Rollings, J.P., Baumeister, A.A., & Baumeister, A.A. The use of overcorrection procedures to eliminate the stereotyped behaviors of retarded individuals. *Behavior Modification*, 1977, *1*, 29–46.

Romanczyk, R.G., & Lockshin, S. *How to create a curriculum for autistic and other handicapped children*. Lawrence, Kans.: H & H Enterprises, 1981.

Rosenblum, S.M., Arick, J.R., Krug, D.A., Stubbs, E.G., Young, N.B., & Pelson, R.O. Auditory brainstem evoked responses in autistic children. *Journal of Autism and Developmental Disorders*, 1980, *10*, 215–225.

Rosenthal, J., Massie, H., & Wulff, K. A comparison of cognitive development in normal and psychotic children in the first two years of life from home movies. *Journal of Autism and Developmental Disorders*, 1980, *10*, 433–444.

Ruder, K.F., & Smith, M.D. Issues in language training. In R.L. Schiefelbusch & L.L. Lloyd (Eds.), *Language perspectives: Acquisition, retardation, and intervention*. Baltimore: University Park Press, 1974.

Rutter, M. Childhood schizophrenia reconsidered. *Journal of Autism and Childhood Schizophrenia*, 1972, *2*, 315–337.

Rutter, M. Diagnosis and definition. In M. Rutter and E. Schopler (Eds.), *Autism: A reappraisal of concepts and treatment*. New York: Plenum Press, 1978. (a)

Rutter, M. Language disorder and infantile autism. In M. Rutter & E. Schopler (Eds.), *Autism: A reappraisal of concepts and treatment*. New York: Plenum Press, 1978. (b)

Rutter, M., & Lockyer, L. A five to fifteen year follow-up study of infantile psychosis. I: Description of the sample. *British Journal of Psychiatry*, 1967, *113*, 1169–1182.

Sailor, W., Guess, D., Goetz, L., Schuler, A., Utley, B., & Baldwin, M. Language and severely handicapped persons: Deciding what to teach to whom. In W. Sailor, B. Wilcox, & L. Brown (Eds.), *Methods of instruction for severely handicapped students*. Baltimore: Paul H. Brooks, 1980.

Salvin, A., Routh, D.K., Foster, R.E., & Lovejoy, K.M. Acquisition of modified American sign language by a mute autistic child. *Journal of Autism and Childhood Schizophrenia*, 1977, *7*, 359–371.

Sanders, D.A. A model for communication. In L.L. Lloyd (Ed.), *Communication assessment and intervention strategies*. Baltimore: University Park Press, 1976.

Schlesinger, I.M. The role of cognitive development and linguistic input in language acquisition. *Journal of Child Language*, 1977, *4*, 153–169.

Schopler, E. *Implementing the mandate for appropriate education of autistic children*. Paper presented at the annual meeting of the National Society for Children and Adults with Autism, Washington, D.C., 1980.

Schopler, E., & Reichler, R.J. Parents as cotherapists in the treatment of psychotic children. *Journal of Autism and Childhood Schizophrenia*, 1971, *1*, 87–102.

Schopler, E., & Reichler, R.J. *Individualized assessment and treatment for autistic and developmentally disabled children. Vol. 1: Psychoeducational profile*. Baltimore: University Park Press, 1979.

Schopler, E., Reichler, R.J., DeVellis, R.F., & Daly, K. Toward objective classification of childhood autism: Childhood Autism Rating Scale (CARS). *Journal of Autism and Developmental Disorders*, 1980, *10*, 91–103.

Schopler, E., Reichler, R.J., & Lansing, M. *Individualized assessment and treatment for autistic and developmentally disabled children. Vol. 2: Teaching strategies for parents and professionals*. Baltimore: University Park Press, 1980.

Schreibman, L., & Lovaas, O.I. Overselective response to social stimuli by autistic children. *Journal of Abnormal Child Psychology*, 1973, *2*, 152–168.

Schuler, A.L. Echolalia: Issues and clinical applications. *Journal of Speech and Hearing Disorders*, 1979, *44*, 411–434.

Schuler, A.L., & Baldwin, M. Nonspeech communication and childhood autism. *Language, Speech, and Hearing Services in Schools*, 1981, *12*, 246–257.

Shane, H.C. Decision making in early augmentative communication system use. In R.L. Schiefelbusch & D.D. Bricker (Eds.), *Early language: Acquisition and intervention*. Baltimore: University Park Press, 1981.

Shearer, T.R., Larson, K., Neuschwander, J., & Gedney, B. Minerals in the hair and nutrient intake of autistic children. *Journal of Autism and Developmental Disorders*, 1982, *12*, 25–34.

Silverman, F.H. *Communication for the speechless*. Englewood Cliffs, N.J.: Prentice-Hall, 1980.

Siple, P., Hatfield, N., & Caccamise, F. The role of visual-perceptual abilities in the acquisition and comprehension of sign language. *American Annals of the Deaf*, 1978, *123*, 852–856.

Sloan, J.L. Differential development of autistic symptoms in a pair of fraternal twins. *Journal of Autism and Childhood Schizophrenia*, 1978, *8*, 191–202.

Sloane, H.N., Johnston, M.K., & Harris, F.R. Remedial procedures for teaching verbal behavior to speech deficient or defective young children. In H.N. Sloane & B. MacAulay (Eds.), *Operant procedures in remedial speech and language training*. Boston: Houghton Mifflin, 1968.

Slobin, D. *Psycholinguistics*. Glenview, Ill.: Scott, Foresman & Co., 1971.

Small, J.G. Sensory evoked responses of autistic children. In D.W. Churchill, G.D. Alpern, & M.K. DeMyer (Eds.), *Infantile autism*. Springfield, Ill.: Charles C Thomas, 1971.

Smith, W.I., & Moore, W.J. *Conditioning and instrumental learning*. New York: McGraw-Hill, 1966.

Spence, M.A. Genetic studies. In E.R. Ritvo (Ed.), *Autism: Diagnosis, current research, and management*. New York: Spectrum Publications, 1976.

Stokoe, W.C. The study and use of sign language. In R.L. Schiefelbusch (Ed.), *Nonspeech language and communication: Analysis and intervention*. Baltimore: University Park Press, 1980.

Stremel, K., & Waryas, C. A behavioral-psycholinguistic approach to language training. In L.V. McReynolds (Ed.), *Developing systematic procedures for training children's language* (American Speech/Language and Hearing Association Monograph No. 18). Washington, D.C.: American Speech/Language and Hearing Association, 1974.

Striefel, S. *Managing behavior. Part 7: Behavioral modification: Teaching a child to imitate*. Lawrence, Kans.: H & H Enterprises, 1974.

Striefel, S., & Owens, C.R. Transfer of stimulus control procedures: Applications to language acquisition training with the developmentally handicapped. *Behavior Research of Severe Developmental Disabilities*, 1980, *1*, 307–331.

Stubbs, E.G. Autistic symptoms in a child with cytomegalo-virus infection. *Journal of Autism and Childhood Schizophrenia*, 1978, *8*, 37–43.

Stubbs, E.G., Crawford, M.L., Burger, D.R., & Vandenbark, A.A. Depressed lymphocyte responsiveness in autistic children. *Journal of Autism and Childhood Schizophrenia*, 1977, *7*, 49–55.

Stubbs, E.G., & Magenis, R.E. HLA and autism. *Journal of Autism and Developmental Disorders*, 1980, *10*, 15–19.

Student, M., & Sohmer, H. Evidence from auditory nerve and brainstem evoked responses for an organic brain lesion in children with autistic traits. *Journal of Autism and Childhood Schizophrenia*, 1978, *8*, 13–19.

Stull, S., Edkins, C., Krause, M., McGavin, G., Brand, L.H., & Webster, C.D. Individual differences in the acquisition of sign language by severely communicatively-impaired children. In C.D. Webster, M.M. Konstantareas, J. Oxman, & J.E. Mack (Eds.), *Autism: New directions in research and education*. New York: Pergamon Press, 1980.

Sulzer-Azaroff, B., & Mayer, G. *Applying behavior analysis procedures with children and youth*. New York: Holt, Rinehart & Winston, 1977.

Sverd, J., Kupietz, S.S., Winsberg, B.G., Hurwic, M.S., & Becker, L. Effects of L-hydroxytryptophan in autistic children. *Journal of Autism and Childhood Schizophrenia*, 1978, *8*, 171–180.

Tager-Flusberg, H. On the nature of linguistic functioning in early infantile autism. *Journal of Autism and Developmental Disorders*, 1981, *11*, 45–56.

Tallal, P. Rapid auditory processing in normal and disordered language development. *Journal of Speech and Hearing Research*, 1976, *19*, 561–571.

Tanguay, P.E. Clinical and electrophysiological research. In E.R. Ritvo (Ed.), *Autism: Diagnosis, current research, and management*. New York: Spectrum Publications, 1976.

Tanguay, P.E. & Edwards, R.M. Electrophysiological studies of autism: The whisper of the bang. *Journal of Autism and Developmental Disorders*, 1982, *12*, 177–185.

Thorpe, W.H. The comparison of vocal communication in animals and man. In R.A. Hinde (Ed.), *Non-vocal communication*. London: Cambridge University Press, 1972.

Thorum, A.R. *Language assessment instruments: Infancy through adulthood*. Springfield, Ill.: Charles C Thomas, 1981.

Torrey, E.F. *Adult schizophrenia as a brain disease: The implications for autism.* Paper presented at the annual meeting of the National Society for Children and Adults with Autism, Washington, D.C., 1980.

Towbin, A. Cerebral dysfunctions related to perinatal damage: Clinical neuropathologic correlations. *Journal of Abnormal Psychology,* 1978, *87,* 617–635.

Tsai, L., Stewart, M.A., & August, G. Implications of sex differences in the familial transmission of infantile autism. *Journal of Autism and Developmental Disorders,* 1981, *11,* 165–173.

Uzgiris, I.C., & Hunt, J.McV. *Assessment in early infancy.* Urbana, Ill.: University of Illinois Press, 1975.

Varmi, J.W., Lovaas, O.I., Koegel, R.L., & Everett, N.L. An analysis of observational learning in autistic and normal children. *Journal of Abnormal Child Psychology,* 1979, *7,* 31–43.

Walker, H.A. Incidence of minor physical anomaly in autism. *Journal of Autism and Childhood Schizophrenia,* 1977, *7,* 165–176.

Walter, W.G., Aldridge, V.J., Cooper, R., O'Gorman, G., McCallum, C., & Winter, A.L. Neurophysiological correlates of apparent defects of sensori-motor integration in autistic children. In D.W. Churchill, G.D. Alpern, & M.K. DeMyer (Eds.), *Infantile Autism.* Springfield, Ill.: Charles C Thomas, 1971.

Watson, D.O. *Talk with your hands* (Vol. 2). Menasha, Wis.: George Banta, 1973.

Watters, R.G., & Watters, W.E. Decreasing self-stimulatory behavior with physical exercise in a group of autistic boys. *Journal of Autism and Developmental Disorders,* 1980, *10,* 379–387.

Weaver, K.S., & Ruder, K.F. The effect of the gestural prompt on syntax training. *Journal of Speech and Hearing Disorders,* 1978, *43,* 513–523.

Weber, D. Toe-walking in children with early childhood autism. *International Journal of Child Psychiatry,* 1978, *43,* 73–83.

Webster, C.D. The characteristics of autism. In C.D. Webster, M.M. Konstantareas, J. Oxman, & J.E. Mack (Eds.), *Autism: New directions in research and education.* New York: Pergamon Press, 1980. (a)

Webster, C.D. Gorky's "Nilushka": Autism case report? *Journal of Autism and Developmental Disorders,* 1980, *10,* 227–229. (b)

Webster, C.F., McPherson, H., Sloman, L., Evans, M.A., & Fruchter, E. Communicating with an autistic boy by gestures. *Journal of Autism and Childhood Schizophrenia,* 1973, *3,* 337–346.

Webster's New Collegiate Dictionary. Springfield, Mass.: G. & C. Merriam, 1981.

Weir, K., & Salisbury, D.M. Acute onset of autistic features following brain damage in a ten-year-old. *Journal of Autism and Developmental Disorders,* 1980, *10,* 185–191.

Wells, K.C., Forehand, R., Hickey, K., & Green, K. Effects of a procedure derived from the overcorrection principle on manipulated and nonmanipulated behaviors. *Journal of Applied Behavior Analysis,* 1977, *10,* 679–687.

Wetherby, A.M., & Gaines, G.H. Cognition and language development in autism. *Journal of Speech and Hearing Disorders,* 1982, *47,* 63–70.

Wetherby, A.M., Koegel, R.L., & Mendal, M. Central auditory nervous system dysfunction in echolalic autistic individuals. *Journal of Speech and Hearing Research,* 1981, *24,* 420–429.

White, O.R. Adaptive performance objectives: Form versus function. In W. Sailor, B. Wilcox, & L. Brown (Eds.), *Methods of instruction for severely handicapped students.* Baltimore: Paul H. Brooks, 1980.

Wing, J.K. Kanner's syndrome: A historical introduction. In L. Wing (Ed.), *Early childhood autism.* New York: Pergamon Press, 1976.

Wing, L. *Autistic children: A guide for parents and professionals.* Secaucus, N.J.: Citadel Press, 1972.

Wing, L. Diagnosis, clinical description and prognosis. In L. Wing (Ed.), *Early childhood autism.* New York: Pergamon Press, 1976.

Wing, L. *Diagnosing autism and autistic-like conditions.* Paper presented at the annual meeting of the National Society for Autistic Children, San Jose, Calif., 1979.

Wing, L. Language, social, and cognitive impairments in autism and severe mental retardation. *Journal of Autism and Developmental Disorders, 1981, 11,* 31–44.

Wolf, D., & Gardner, H. On the structure of early symbolization. In R.L. Schiefelbusch & D.D. Bricker (Eds.), *Early language: Acquisition and intervention.* Baltimore: University Park Press, 1981.

Wolf, M.M., Risley, T., & Mees, H. Application of operant conditioning procedures to the behavior problems of an autistic child. *Behavioral Research and Therapy, 1964, 1,* 305–312.

Young, J.G., Kyprie, R.M., Ross, N.T., & Cohen, D.J. Serum dopamine-beta-hydroxylase activity: Clinical applications in child psychiatry. *Journal of Autism and Developmental Disorders, 1980, 10,* 1–14.

Yuwiler, A., Geller, E., & Ritvo, E.R. Neurobiochemical research. In E.R. Ritvo (Ed.), *Autism: Diagnosis, current research, and management.* New York: Spectrum Publications, 1976.

Zifferblatt, S.M., Burton, S.D., Horner, R., & White, T. Establishing generalization effects among autistic children. *Journal of Autism and Schizophrenia, 1977, 7,* 337–347.

Appendix A

Sample Behavior Management Forms

The following sample forms are provided for use by teachers and therapists in managing the behavior of autistic children, as discussed in Chapter 3.

Baseline Chart

Target Behavior:

Baseline:

Time:	9:00	10:00	11:00	12:00	1:00	2:00	3:00	Total
Activity:								
Monday								
Tuesday								
Wednesday								
Thursday								
Friday								

Total for week:

Chart for Recording Behavioral Change

BEHAVIOR CHANGE CHART									
Target Behavior:									
Baseline:									
Consequence:									
Time									
Activity									
Date									Total

Behavior Change Graph

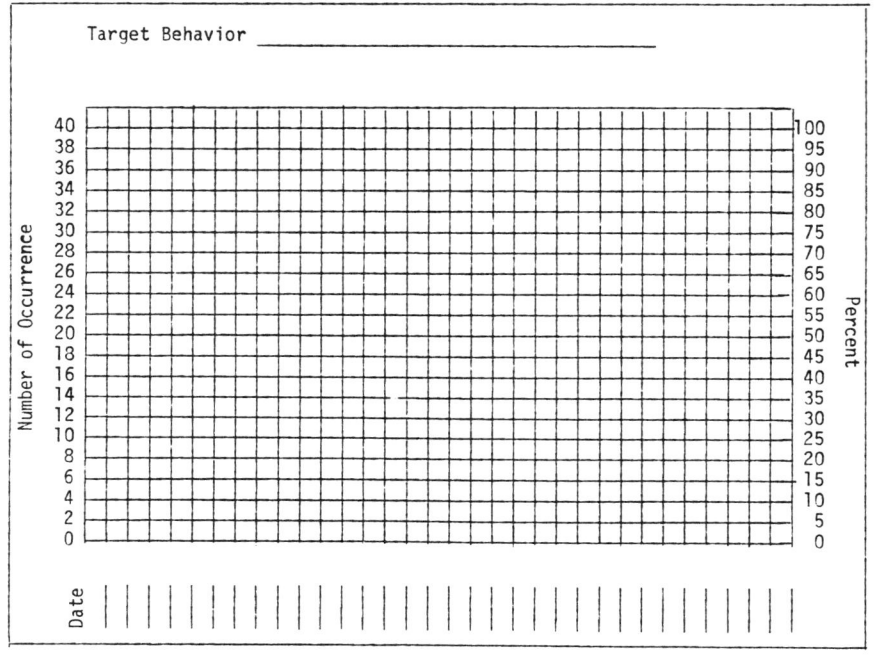

Sample Form for Recording Discrete Trial Data

The following sample form is provided for use by teachers and therapists in recording data from discrete trial programs, as discussed in Chapter 5.

Discrete Trial Data Sheet

PROGRAM:

Date: ___ % Correct ___

(Discrete trial data sheet form with a grid of cells, each labeled "Date:" and "% Correct ___")

Sample Program Form

The following sample form is provided for use by teachers and therapists in implementing attending programs (Chapter 5), imitation and manual communication programs (Chapter 6), and manual communication programs using overcorrection (Chapter 7).

Program Instruction Form

Program: _____

Goal:

Setting:

Materials:

Criterion for mastery:

Procedures for the delivery of consequences:

    Reinforcement:

    Punishment:

Activities:

PROGRAM:

Program Activities Data Form

Stimulus	Prompt	Response	Consequence	Data
				Session 1: Date _____ % Correct _____
				Session 2: Date _____ % Correct _____
				Session 3: Date _____ % Correct _____
				Session 4: Date _____ % Correct _____

Index

compulsive, 1-5
deficits and excesses of, 38-39
diagnosis of, 15-20
disturbed, 1
extinction of, 46-54
and imitation training, 121-135
and learning tasks, 77-79
management of, 37-58, 189-192
measurement of, 54-57
modeling of, 148-150
modification of, 11-12, 15
normal echolalic, 27-28
operant conditioning of, 4
overcorrection procedures for,
   59-68
and parent training, 165-166
prerequisite, 105-106
programming of new, 57
recording of, 190-192
reinforcement of, 41-44
ritualistic, 1-5, 9
target, 38-53
vocal, 103
Behavior management. *See* Behavior
Biochemistry, and autism, 12-15
Blissymbolics, 112-114
Body movements. *See* Motor
   responses
Brain chemistry, and autism, 12-14
Brain damage, 5-14

C

Case studies. *See* Studies
Causes, of autism, 12-15
Central nervous system, 8, 10
Charts, for behavior management,
   190-192
Checklist, for autism screening,
   19-20
Chromosomes, and autism, 15
Classification, of autism, 7
Classroom, manual for, 20
Clinicians, speech, 164

Clothing, aversion to, 9
Cognition
   and autism, 4
   deficits in, 33-34
Cognitive scales, 18
Communication
   See also Nonverbal communication
   boards, 112-114
   deviant, 30-31
   gestural, 111-114
   impairment in, 6
   manual, 126-135, 137-140, 195
   modes of, 103-104
   overcorrection in teaching, 137-162
   signing as, 114-118
   teaching of, 103-120
   training manual for, 20
   visual, 111-120
Congenital diseases, and autism, 12
Consequences
   See also Reinforcement
   in attending training, 73, 76
Criteria
   for attending programs, 76
   for autism, 5-7, 15-20
Curriculum
   for communication programs, 20,
      107-120
Cytomegalovirus, 12

D

Data
   in attending trials, 74-75
   collection of, 54
   recording of, 189-196
Deafness
   examinations for, 107
   manual communication for,
      115-119
Development
   abnormal paralinguistic, 31-33
   disturbances of, 6, 30-31
   and echolalia, 27

Skills
  See also Motor responses
  acquisition of, 108
  emerging, 19
  evaluation of, 104-107
  goals for, 164-165
  mastery of, 137-140
  parental training of, 166
  and PEP assessment, 18
  prelinguistic, 33
  programming of, 57
  self-help, 38
  and social development, 11-15, 31
Sleep patterns, 10
Social development, and autism, 1-21
Social imitation, 7
Social levels, 106
Social skills. *See* Skills
Social withdrawal, 8
Social workers, role of, 164
Special education teachers, 164
Speech
  See also Language
  abnormal melody, 7
  of autistic children, 2-4, 24-28
  as language manifestation, 103
  manual communication and, 115-119
  pathologist's role, 164
  prelanguage skills, 7
  as prognostic indicator, 11-12
  programs for development of, 107
Standard test procedures, 105
Startle response, 48
Statistics, on autism, 11
Stimulus
  in discrete trials, 72-73
  in overcorrection program, 153-162
  visual, 112-114
Strategies
  for the classroom, 20
  for managing at home, 167-169
Structure, use of, 69-71
Studies
  of autism, 1-21

  of manual communication, 114-118
  of overcorrection, 138-140
  of parental roles, 163
Successive approximations, 46
Symbolization, 33
Symbols
  American sign language, 115-116
  gestural, 115-119
  and language, 103, 112
  manual communication program and, 126-135
Symptoms, of autism, 1-21
Syndrome
  of autism, 4-5
  disease, 10
Syntactic rules, 104
Systems
  of communication, 103-120, 126-135
  of manual signing, 114-118

T

Tactile perception, 9-10
Tantrums, 105
Target behaviors, 38-53
Tasks
  analysis of, 57, 72-73
  verbal and motor imitation, 146
Teaching
  of attending, 69-71
  autistic children, 16
  and control, 44
  environments for, 71-72, 167-169
  individualized, 19, 164
  overcorrection in, 137-162
  of parents, 166-167
  and pupil ratios, 78, 168
  reinforcement and, 44, 59
  skills of, 38
  by successive approximation, 46
Techniques, behavioral management, 20

About the Author

PAIGE S. HINERMAN, M.S., received her master of science degree in speech pathology from the University of Utah and is currently earning her doctorate degree. She has worked with autistic children and their parents for nine years. As a therapist and classroom supervisor at the Children's Behavior Therapy Unit in Salt Lake City, Utah, she has worked with autistic, behaviorally disturbed, language-disordered, and mentally retarded children. As an adjunct clinical instructor at the University of Utah, she has supervised graduate students in the department of speech pathology and audiology. She has been director of the Utah Program for Autistic Children, a federal demonstration project involving a group home for young autistic children.